Lectures in
Cardiovascular
Physiology

Lectures in
Cardiovascular
Physiology

K Sri Nageswari MD FABMS

Professor
Department of Physiology
Dr VRK Women's Medical College
Hyderabad

International Fellow in Medical Education
Ex-Professor and Head
Department of Physiology
Government Medical College
Chandigarh

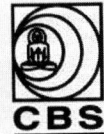

CBS

CBS Publishers & Distributors Pvt Ltd

New Delhi • Bengaluru • Chennai • Kochi • Kolkata • Mumbai
Hyderabad • Jharkhand • Nagpur • Patna • Pune • Uttarakhand

Lectures in
Cardiovascular Physiology

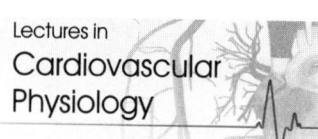

ISBN: 978-93-86827-92-0

Copyright © Author and Publisher

First Edition: 2018

Published by Satish Kumar Jain and produced by Varun Jain for

CBS Publishers & Distributors Pvt Ltd

4819/XI Prahlad Street, 24 Ansari Road, Daryaganj, New Delhi 110 002, India.
Ph: 23289259, 23266861, 23266867   Website: www.cbspd.com
Fax: 011-23243014   e-mail: delhi@cbspd.com; cbspubs@airtelmail.in.
Corporate Office: 204 FIE, Industrial Area, Patparganj, Delhi 110 092
Ph: 4934 4934   Fax: 4934 4935   e-mail: publishing@cbspd.com; publicity@cbspd.com

Branches

- **Bengaluru:** Seema House 2975, 17th Cross, K.R. Road,
  Banasankari 2nd Stage, Bengaluru 560 070, Karnataka
  Ph: +91-80-26771678/79   Fax: +91-80-26771680   e-mail: bangalore@cbspd.com
- **Chennai:** 7, Subbaraya Street, Shenoy Nagar, Chennai 600 030, Tamil Nadu
  Ph: +91-44-26680620, 26681266   Fax: +91-44-42032115   e-mail: chennai@cbspd.com
- **Kochi:** Ashana House, No. 39/1904, AM Thomas Road, Valanjambalam,
  Ernakulam 682 016, Kochi, Kerala
  Ph: +91-484-4059061-65   Fax: +91-484-4059065   e-mail: kochi@cbspd.com
- **Kolkata:** 6/B, Ground Floor, Rameswar Shaw Road, Kolkata-700 014, West Bengal
  Ph: +91-33-22891126, 22891127, 22891128   e-mail: kolkata@cbspd.com
- **Mumbai:** 83-C, Dr E Moses Road, Worli, Mumbai-400018, Maharashtra
  Ph: +91-22-24902340/41   Fax: +91-22-24902342   e-mail: mumbai@cbspd.com

Representatives

- **Hyderabad**   0-9885175004   • **Jharkhand**   0-9811541605   • **Nagpur**   0-9021734563
- **Patna**   0-9334159340   • **Pune**   0-9623451994   • **Uttarakhand**   0-9716462459

Printed at India Binding House, Noida, UP, India

to
My husband, Dr KR Sarma
For the compromises he made in ensuring
the realisation of my dreams
My six children, Sharat–Sunita, Ravi–Raji, Aarati–Ram
For their abundant love and affection
My parents, late Major VS Rao and Mrs Lakshmi
For bringing me into this world
Last but not the least
To all the first year medical students of this wonderful country
For whom I have prepared the book
Lectures in Cardiovascular Physiology

Preface

Lectures in Cardiovascular Physiology is an adjunct to the standard textbooks of physiology describing cardiovascular physiology in nutshell. The lecture notes describe in concise manner various physiological phenomena, enumerating the salient features in the form of flowcharts and block diagrams for better comprehension. The lectures are meant for the students of MBBS and allied disciplines. It is difficult for the students to read the entire textbook prior to the examinations and there is paucity of time. This book is written with the intention to help the student in preparing for the theory and viva-voce examinations and for easy revision and memorisation of the salient features, after going through standard textbooks. These lectures are also useful while preparing for various entrance examinations. Though the lectures are not a complete replacement for the standard textbooks of physiology describing the cardiovascular system in detail, care was taken to describe all the chapters falling under the heading of cardiovascular physiology with minute details. The figures are less in number as compared to standard textbooks. The lecture notes were being distributed to undergraduate medical students during the past few years and as per their feedback, have been excellent in clearing their concepts, understanding and memorisation of the subject of physiology.

The author acknowledges the secretarial assistance provided by Ms Parminder Kaur and the Department of Medicine, Government Medical College and Hospital, Chandigarh for providing ECG tracings.

K Sri Nageswari

Contents

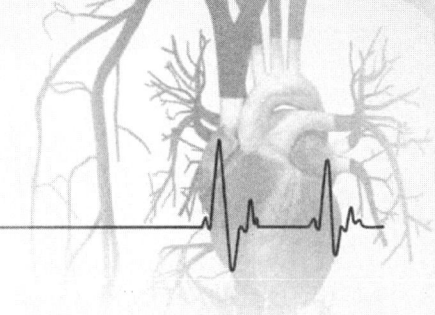

1

Heart and Blood Vessels

Cardiovascular system is one of the major coordinating and integrating systems of the body. It consists of heart and blood vessels.

HEART

- Right side of the heart
- Left side of the heart
- Layers of the wall of the heart
- Septa of the heart
- Valves of the heart

BLOOD VESSELS

- Arterial system
- Venous system

CIRCULATION AND ITS DIVISIONS

- Systemic circulation
- Pulmonary circulation

Flow of blood through heart is unidirectional.

FUNCTIONS OF CIRCULATORY SYSTEM

1. To supply O_2, nutrients and essential substances to the tissues of the body
2. Remove end products from tissues

3. Maintenance of fluid balance
4. Regulation of body temperature
5. Distribution of hormones, drugs, etc.

MORPHOLOGICAL STRUCTURE OF THE HEART

Right side of the heart consists of right atrium and right ventricle. It pumps blood through the pulmonary artery to the lungs. It has got the pacemaker, the SA node in the right atrium that originates the cardiac impulse and AV node that conducts these impulses to the ventricles. It has superior vena cava that brings the deoxygenated blood from the head and neck and upper limbs and inferior vena cava that brings the deoxygenated blood from lower parts of body. Right atrium opens into the right ventricle through the tricuspid valve (flap valves). Pulmonary artery carries deoxygenated blood that is pumped into lungs by right ventricle.

Left side of the heart consists of left atrium and left ventricle. Left atrium opens into the left ventricle through the mitral valve (bicuspid valve) and empties the oxygenated blood into the left ventricle through this. Left ventricle pumps oxygenated blood through systemic aorta throughout the body. As cardiac pumping is intermittent, continuous flow is maintained by elastic recoil of the aorta.

Layers

Outer fibrous layer is known as *pericardium*. It is similar to tunica adventitia of large vessels. Fibrous layer protects the heart from overstretching.

Inner serous layer is divided into:
Outer—parietal pericardium
Inner—visceral pericardium

In between the parietal and visceral pericardium, the pericardial space has thin film of fluid.

Myocardium

Middle layer is formed by cardiac muscle cells or fibres. Three types of muscle fibres are:

1. *Muscle fibres that form the contractile unit of the heart*

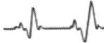

2. *Muscle fibres that form the pacemaker that initiates the impulses for contraction of the heart*
3. *Muscle fibres that form the conductive system of the heart through which impulses are conducted*

Muscle Fibres Forming Contractile Unit

These muscle fibres are striated, are similar to skeletal muscle, but are involuntary. The lattice work is formed by the muscle fibres dividing, then recombining and then spreading again. Cardiac muscle acts as a syncytium. The dark areas are known as intercalated discs. These are cell membranes that separate individual cardiac muscle cells from one another. Many individual cardiac muscle cells are connected in series with each other. Electrical resistance through the intercalated discs is 1/400th of the resistance through the outside membrane of the cardiac muscle fibre.

Muscle Fibres Forming Pacemaker

Some muscle fibres of the heart are modified into a specialised structure namely pacemaker. These muscle fibres have less striations.

Pacemaker

SA node is formed of pacemaker cells (P cells) situated in the posterior wall of the right atrium near the opening of the superior vena cava.

Muscle Fibres Forming Conductive System

They are modified specialised cells, also known as junctional tissues. They conduct the impulses rapidly from SA node through internodal fibres, AV node, bundle of His, branches of bundle of His and Purkinje fibres to ventricles.

Endocardium

It is the innermost layer of the heart wall. It is thin, smooth and glistening membrane formed by single layer of endothelial cells that continues as endothelium of the blood vessels.

Septa of the Heart

The two atria are separated by interatrial septum which is fibrous. The two ventricles are separated by interventricular septum which has upper membranous part and lower muscular part.

Valves of the Heart

They permit the flow of blood through the heart in only one direction. They are atrioventricular valves and semilunar valves.

Atrioventricular Valves

On the left side of the heart, between the left atrium and left ventricle, it is known as *mitral valve* that has 2 cusps or flaps. On the right side, between the right atrium and right ventricle the *tricuspid valve* has 3 cusps. Brim of the valves is attached to the atrioventricular ring, which is the fibrous connection between atria and ventricles that allows the atria and ventricles to function separately as syncytia. Cusps are attached to the papillary muscles by means of structures known as *chordae tendineae*. Papillary muscles arise from inner aspect of the ventricles. Papillary muscles play important role in closure of the cusps and prevent back flow of blood from ventricle to atria during ventricular contraction.

Semilunar Valves

Semilunar valves are present at the openings of systemic aorta and pulmonary artery and are known as *aortic and pulmonary valve*, respectively. These consist of three flaps each and open towards the aorta/pulmonary artery and prevent backflow of blood into the ventricles.

BLOOD VESSELS

Aorta

Aorta arises from left ventricle and is predominantly an elastic structure, i.e. ratio of elastic to smooth muscle is greatest. It is also known as *windkessel vessel* due to the property of elastic recoil during diastole. The cross-sectional area of the aorta is 2.5 cm^2 and has the maximum velocity of blood flow as 33 cm/sec. The aorta and arteries have 13 per cent of the total blood volume. With pulsatile pumping of the heart, the arterial pressure is maximum in the aorta. The systolic pressure in the aorta is 120 mmHg and diastolic pressure is 80 mmHg.

Arteries (Large, Medium and Small)

Arteries are muscular. The large arteries offer little frictional resistance and hence the pressure drop across them is not much. The pressure drop is greatest in the small arteries and arterioles. The cross-sectional area of small arteries is 20 cm^2. Blood flows with a high velocity through the arteries.

Arterioles

Arterioles vessels are highly muscular and they offer great frictional resistance to blood flow. Hence the pressure drop across these vessels is greatest (35 mmHg). They act as stop-cocks and regulate blood flow in the tissues. These are known as *resistance vessels*. Along with capillaries, they have 7 per cent of total blood volume and the cross-sectional area is 40 cm^2. The muscular layers of the arterioles have noradrenergic fibres which cause vasoconstriction. Small changes in the caliber of the vessels cause large changes in resistance.

Capillaries

The capillaries have thin walls consisting of single layer of endothelium. They are the vessels where exchange of nutrients, fluids, gases, electrolytes, drugs, hormones and other substances takes place. The pulsatile arterial blood flow resulting from intermittent ejection of blood from the heart is converted to steady flow by the time blood reaches capillaries. This is due to damping caused by distensibility of arteries and frictional resistance in the small arteries and arterioles. The cross-sectional area of the capillaries is maximum, i.e. 2500 cm^2. The arterial pressure at arteriolar ends of the capillaries is 35 mmHg and at venous ends it is 10 mmHg. The velocity of blood flow is the

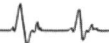
lowest in the capillaries at 0.3 mm/sec. Thus blood remains only for a short duration of 1 to 3 seconds in the capillaries during which the exchange takes place.

Veins and Venules

Out of the total blood volume, 84 per cent is in systemic circulation and 64 per cent of this volume is in the venous system. The arterial pressure drops to 0 mmHg in the venous system. The cross-sectional areas of venules, small veins and venae cavae are 250, 80 and 8 cm², respectively. The veins are known as *capacitance vessels* as they function as reservoirs.

Pulmonary Artery and Pulmonary Vein

Pulmonary circulation is also known as lesser circulation. It has 9 per cent of total blood volume. The pressure in pulmonary artery is 25 mmHg during systole and 8 mmHg during diastole and the mean pulmonary arterial pressure is 16 mmHg. The heart contains 7 per cent of the blood volume.

2

Cardiac Electrophysiology

DEFINITIONS

Membrane Potential

It represents the voltage difference between the inside of the cell and the surrounding extracellular environment of the cell, i.e. interstitial tissue.

Resting Membrane Potential

The cell membrane is polarised at rest. There is a steady potential difference between the interior and the exterior of the cell at rest, which is known as *resting membrane potential*. This steady state continues till it is supervened by action potential.

Depolarisation

With activity, the polarity reverses and the inside of the cell becomes more positive.

Repolarisation

Following depolarisation inside of the cell becomes negative, i.e. restoration of normal resting potential occurs and "Status quo" continues.

Hyperpolarisation

Inside of the cell becomes more negative, i.e. the polarisation of the membrane increases.

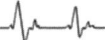

ELECTRICAL ACTIVITY OF THE HEART

Two centuries ago, Galvani (1737–1798) and Volta (1745–1827) stated that electrical phenomena were involved in spontaneous contractions of the heart.

Kollicker and Muller (1856) placed nerve of an innervated skeletal muscle in contact with beating frog's heart, and the skeletal muscle contracted.

Conclusion

- Spontaneous excitation of the heart occurs
- Sufficient electrical activity is generated in the heart during activity
- When placed in contact with beating heart, motor nerve fibres got excited, leading to stimulation of skeletal muscle, resulting in contraction of skeletal muscle

Resting Membrane Potential (Vm)

The interior of the resting cardiac muscle cell is 90 mV negative to the exterior.

Action Potential

When the cardiac muscle cell is stimulated electrically, the potential difference is reversed and goes up to +20 mV to + 30 mV. The action potential is divided into the following parts:

Phase 0 – Rapid upstroke

Phase 1 – Brief period of early repolarisation

Phase 2 – Plateau

Phase 3 – Repolarisation

Phase 4 – State of polarisation

Completion of repolarisation coincides with peak force. Two types of action potentials occur in cardiac muscle.

Fast Response

It occurs in atrial and ventricular myocytes and Purkinje fibres of the heart. Upstroke is faster and the amplitude and extent of the action potential are greater.

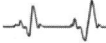

Slow Response

It occurs in SA node, the pacemaker of the heart and AV node. These are specialized junctional tissues of the heart. SA node originates the rhythm of the heart and AV node conducts the impulse from atria to ventricles. The upstroke is slow, amplitude and the extent of the action potential are less and the fibres are more liable for conduction blocks.

IONIC BASIS OF RESTING MEMBRANE POTENTIAL

Various phases of cardiac action potential are associated with changes in permeability of the cell membrane to Na^+, K^+ and Ca^{2+} ions.

Net diffusion of an ion depends on:
• Permeability of the membrane for that particular ion
• Transmembrane concentration difference
• Transmembrane electrical potential difference

Resting membrane is more permeable to K^+. The electrostatic and chemical gradients for K^+ are directed inward and outward, respectively. K^+ diffuses out through specific K^+ channels. One of the specific K^+ channels is a voltage regulated channel that conducts inwardly rectifying K^+ current (i_{K1}).

IONIC BASIS OF FAST RESPONSE

Phase 0

With stimulus, resting membrane potential is disturbed. When it is changed to a critical value (threshold) of –65 mV, fast Na^+ channels open and rapid depolarisation occurs. These channels can be blocked by tetrodotoxin. Overshoot reaches an amplitude of +20 to +30 mV.

Two types of gates operate:
• M gate—activation gate, opens the channel at –65 mV
• H gate—inactivation gate, closes the channel at +30 mV. Na^+ entry ceases.

Phase 1

Early brief period of repolarisation represented by notch between end of upstroke and beginning of plateau. This is due to

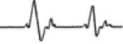

activation of K^+ channels known as "Transient outward current (ito)". K^+ efflux occurs.

Phase 2

Genesis of plateau: Ca^{2+} enters through Ca^{2+} channels (L-type channels). Activation and inactivation are slow. Influx of Ca^{2+} (positive charge) is counterbalanced by efflux of K^+ (positive charge) through i_{to}, i_K and i_{K1} potassium ion channels. Influx of Ca^{2+} into the cell throughout the plateau is involved in excitation-contraction coupling.

Calcium conductance (gCa) is enhanced by:
1. Norepinephrine (α adrenergic receptor agonist)
2. Isoproterenol (β adrenergic receptor agonist)
3. Other catecholamines

Calcium conductance is reduced by:

Acetylcholine: K^+ conductance during plateau: Both the chemical and electrostatic forces favour efflux of K^+. However, potassium conductance (g_K) decreases as Vm (membrane potential)attains positive values near the peak of the upstroke. Reduction in g_K at positive and low negative values is called *inward rectification*, which is characteristic of i_{K1} current. Another K^+ channel, the *delayed rectifier (i_K) channel*, also contributes to plateau. Delayed rectifier channels are activated very slowly (by the end of phase 2) and play minor role during phase 2. They increase g_K and they contribute to final repolarisation in phase 3.

Phase 3

Genesis of final repolarisation: Efflux of K^+ exceeds influx of Ca^{2+} through three outward K^+ currents—i_{to}, i_K, i_{K1}. The i_{to} and i_K channels help initiate repolarisation. When the outward K^+ current exceeds inward Ca^{2+} current, repolarisation begins. Inwardly rectifying current (i_{K1}) contributes substantially once phase 3 has been initiated.

Phase 4

Restoration of ionic concentrations: Excess Na^+ that entered during phase 0 and throughout the cardiac cycle is eliminated through Na^+, K^+ -ATPase. 3 Na^+ are extruded in exchange for $2K^+$. Excess

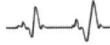

Ca^{2+} that entered through phase 2 is removed by Na^+/Ca^{2+} exchanger, which pumps in $3Na^+$ for $1Ca^{2+}$. Ca^{2+} is also driven out by ATP driven Ca^{2+} pump.

IONIC BASIS OF SLOW RESPONSE

Slow response occurs in SA node and AV node. Upstroke is less steep, phase 1 is absent, plateau is less prolonged and transition from plateau to final repolarisation is less distinct. Blocking the fast Na^+ channels with tetrodotoxin converts the fast response to slow response.

Depolarisation: Occurs due to influx of Ca^{2+} through Ca^{2+} channels.

Repolarisation: Due to increased K^+ conductance through i_{K1} and i_K channels.

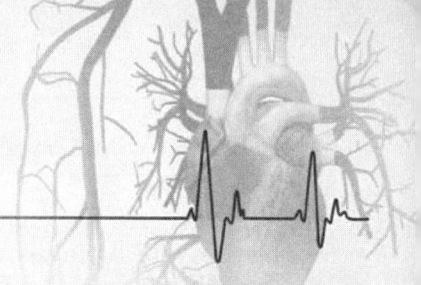

3

Properties of the Heart

1. *Automaticity*: It is the ability of a tissue to originate or initiate its own impulse or beat, e.g. pacemaker activity of SA node.
2. *Rhythmicity*: The regular/rhythmic nature of pacemaker activity.
3. *Excitability*: The ability of the heart to respond to a given stimulus.
4. *Conductivity*: Ability to conduct the impulse from the site of its origin, i.e. from SA node, through specialised conductive system of the heart to the atria and ventricles is known as conductivity.
5. *Contractility*: Ability of the tissue to shorten in length (contract), in response to a stimulus is called contractility.
6. *All or none law*: When a stimulus of either threshold intensity or above threshold intensity is applied, the heart muscle responds to the maximum. If the stimulus is of below threshold intensity, it does not respond at all.
7. *Refractory period*: It is the interval of time during which a normal cardiac impulse cannot re-excite an already excited area of cardiac muscle. The heart muscle cannot be tetanised due to this property.

Self excitation forms the basis of automaticity and rhythmicity and is the special property of the junctional and conductive systems of the heart.

1. *SA node or sinoatrial node*: The normal rhythmical impulse is originated here.

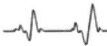

2. *Internodal pathways*: Conduct impulse from SA node to AV node.
3. *AV node or atrioventricular node*: The impulse from the atria is delayed here before passing onto ventricles.
4. *AV bundle*: Conducts the impulse from atria into ventricles. It originates from AV node and divides into two branches.
5. *The left and right bundles of Purkinje fibres*: These conduct cardiac impulse to all parts of the ventricles.

SINOATRIAL NODE (SA NODE)

It is a small, flattened ellipsoid strip of tissue, located in the superior posterior wall of right atrium, below and lateral to the opening of superior vena cava. The SA nodal fibres are 3–5 µm in width, have no contractile elements and connect directly with the atrial muscle fibres. Thus the action potential spreads directly to atrial muscle fibres. Sinoatrial node is the pacemaker of the heart. The discharge rate of SA node is 70–80/minute. Being the fastest, it dictates the rhythm of the heart.

• Discharge rate of AV node is 40–60/minute.
• Discharge rate of Purkinje fibres is 15–40/minute.

IONIC BASIS OF AUTOMATICITY AND PACEMAKER POTENTIAL

When the membrane potential becomes more negative than –50 mV, slow diastolic depolarisation occurs in the pacemaker cells of SA node.

Three ionic currents are responsible:
1. An inward Na^+ current, i_f (funny current)
2. An inward Ca^{2+} current, i_{Ca}
3. An outward K^+ current, i_K

1. *Funny current (i_f)*: Inward Na^+ movement through specific Na^+ channels occurs at the completion of repolarisation, as the membrane potential becomes negative, about –50 mV. These channels are different from the fast Na^+ channels.
2. *Inward Ca^{2+} current (i_{Ca})*: It is activated at the end of phase 4 when transmembrane potential reaches a value of –55 mV. Ca^{2+} channels are activated and influx of Ca^{2+}

into the cell increases that leads to upstroke of the action potential. Decrease in external Ca^{2+} concentration and Ca^{2+} channel blockers result in decreased amplitude and decreased slope of diastolic depolarisation.

3. *Delayed rectifier current (i_K):* Efflux of K^+ opposes the diastolic depolarisation by the two inward currents. After the upstroke of the action potential, K^+ efflux repolarises the cell. K^+ efflux continues beyond maximal repolarisation but diminishes throughout phase 4.

Adrenergic transmitters augment all the three ionic currents involved in automaticity (augmentations of i_f and i_{Ca} exceed the enhancement of i_K). Acetylcholine causes hyperpolarisation by decreased i_f and i_{Ca} currents and increased efflux of K^+ through acetylcholine regulated K^+ channels.

TRANSMISSION OF CARDIAC IMPULSE

Conduction Through Atria

1. Direct spread of impulse through the atria at the rate of 0.3 m/sec.
2. *Internodal pathways:* Anterior, middle and posterior internodal pathways consist of specialized conduction fibres that conduct at the rate of 1 m/sec. They terminate in AV node. It takes 0.03 sec for the impulse to reach AV node.
3. Anterior interatrial band passes from right to left atrium and conduction takes place through this.

AV Node

It is located immediately behind the tricuspid valve, in the posterior wall of right atrium. There is a delay of 0.09 seconds in transmission of impulse in AV node and a further delay of 0.04 seconds occurs in the penetrating portion of the AV bundle. Total delay of 0.16 seconds occurs up to this point, after origin of impulse in SA node.

Advantage

The delay allows time for the atria to empty their contents (blood) into ventricles.

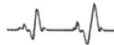

Cause for the delay
1. Small size of the fibres
2. Less number of gap junctions, hence great resistance to movement of ions.

Purkinje System

Rapid transmission, 1.5–4 m/sec, fibres are larger than ventricular muscle fibres, high level of permeability of gap junctions at the intercalated discs.

Left and Right Bundle Branches

AV bundle penetrates the fibrous tissue (penetrating portion), passes downward for 5 to 15 mm in the ventricular septum towards the apex, divides into left and right bundle branches which spread downwards, course around each ventricle and back towards the base. The Purkinje fibres penetrate about one-third of the muscle mass. Impulse transmission takes 0.03 seconds in the Purkinje system.

Ventricular Muscle

Arranged like a double spiral, with fibrous septa in between, the impulse angulates towards the surface, in the direction of spirals. The velocity of transmission is 0.3 to 0.5 m/sec. Time taken for transmission from endocardial to epicardial surface is 0.03 seconds.

Abnormal Pacemakers

Ectopic pacemaker: Some other part of the heart discharges at a faster rate than the SA node and dictates the rhythm of the heart under abnormal conditions.
1. AV node
2. Purkinje fibres or rarely a portion of atrial or ventricular muscle.

Causes
1. Abnormality in any one of the above structures
2. Conduction blocks, e.g. AV block

REFRACTORY PERIOD OF CARDIAC MUSCLE

The absolute refractory period of the ventricle is 0.25–0.3 seconds, during which the cardiac muscle does not respond to restimulation. There is additional relative refractory period of 0.05 seconds during which heart muscle can be excited by very strong excitatory stimulus. In the atria, the refractory period is 0.15 seconds.

4

Excitation–Contraction Coupling

In cardiac muscle, the action potential travels along the sarcolemma and then into the muscle fibre, through the T-tubules that invaginate the cardiac fibres at Z lines. Depolarisation of the T-tubular system evokes Ca^{2+} release from a specialised membrane bound organelle, the *sacroplasmic reticulum*. Ca^{2+} enters through the Ca^{2+} channels in the sarcolemma of cardiac muscle fibre and T-tubules during the plateau phase of action potential. The released Ca^{2+} causes a sudden increase in cytosolic free Ca^{2+}.

The amount of calcium that enters the myocardial cell during depolarisation is not sufficient to induce contraction. However, it acts as a trigger to release stored Ca^{2+} from sacroplasmic reticulum (Ca^{2+} induced Ca^{2+} release). The intracellular Ca^{2+} ($10^{-7}M - 10^{-6}M$) increases to $10^{-5}M$ during excitation (extracellular Ca^{2+} concentration is $10^{-3}M$).

The following factors increase the Ca^{2+} concentration inside the myocardial cell, and hence the developed force.

By increasing the external Ca^{2+} concentration or decreasing the extracellular Na^+ concentration, the Na^+ gradient is reversed and less of Ca^{2+} is pumped out of the cell by the Na^+/Ca^{2+} exchanger (Na^+/Ca^{2+} exchanger pumps Ca^{2+} that has entered the cell during depolarisation, out of the cell, in exchange for Na^+). When the extracellular Ca^{2+} concentration is increased, less Ca^{2+} is pumped out of the cell.

On the other hand, decrease in extracellular Ca^{2+} concentration or increase in extracellular Na^+/Na^+ gradient across sacrolemma cause decrease in the tension developed by myocardial cell.

Excitation–Contraction Coupling

The primary structures at which excitation–contraction coupling (E-C coupling) occurs consist of T-tubules flanked by sarcoplasmic reticulum terminal cisternae.

The two key proteins involved in excitation–contraction coupling:
1. The dihydropyridine receptors (DHPRs) are found in the T-tubules.
2. The ryanodine receptor(RyR) is found in the membrane of sarcoplasmic reticulum.

The DHPRs and RyRs are calcium channels and are responsible for increasing the Ca^{2+} concentration inside the cell. Dihydropyridines are drugs that block T-tubule calcium channels (e.g. nifedipine). The L-type voltage-gated calcium channels are often referred to as dihydropyridine receptors. Ryanodine is a plant alkaloid that binds to RyRs.

ROLE OF CELLULAR Ca²⁺ DURING VENTRICULAR SYSTOLE AND DIASTOLE

Ventricular Systole

Pacemaker originates activating currents → conduction through the ventricle → activating currents spread through sarcolemma of myocardial cell and T-tubules → Ca^{2+} enters during plateau phase of action potential through sarcolemma (Ca^{2+} channels) and T-tubules (dihydropyridine receptors) → Ca^{2+} binds to ryanodine receptors intracellularly and acts as a trigger for release of stored Ca^{2+} → increase in intracellular Ca^{2+} (from 0.1 to 1 µM) → Ca^{2+} binds to troponin C → inhibition by troponin I is released → tropomyosin moves in a switch-like motion on actin, exposing the active sites on actin filament → myosin cross-bridges bind to actin → binding of myosin cross-bridges to active sites on actin filaments also facilitates the neighbouring cross-bridges (cooperative activation) → actin filaments slide towards centre of sarcomere → tension/force is developed by myocardial cell.

The muscle cell tension is determined by the number of actin-cross-bridge interactions.

→ leading to

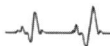

This in turn is determined by:
1. The sarcomere length (preload)
2. The load to be lifted and shortening velocity (afterload which is aortic pressure in case of left ventricle)
3. Availability of Ca^{2+} and relative activation of thin filament as determined by the saturation of troponin with Ca^{2+} (contractility)

In resting physiological states, only 25 per cent of cross-bridges are activated by the Ca^{2+} released from sacroplasmic reticulum. With each cross-bridge cycling, one molecule of ATP is split.

The following events occur at the end of systole:
1. Ca^{2+} influx and Ca^{2+} release from sacroplasmic reticulum stop.
2. Sacroplasmic reticulum takes up Ca^{2+} through ATP driven Ca^{2+} pump. CyclicAMP dependent protein kinase phosphorylates a protein, *Phospholamban,* which stimulates Ca^{2+} pump.
3. Phosphorylation of troponin I inhibits binding of Ca^{2+} to troponin C.→ tropomyosin blocks the interactive sites of actin and myosin filaments thus blocking the cyclic reaction of myosin cross-bridges with actin. Ventricular diastole occurs.

Energy consuming mechanisms of myocardial cell:
1. With each cross-bridge cycle, one ATP molecule is split (myosin ATPase)
2. Na^+/K^+ pump
3. Sacroplasmic reticulum Ca^{2+} pump
4. Ca^{2+} pump of the cell membrane

PRESSURE DEVELOPMENT IN LEFT VENTRICLE

For cardiac contraction, preload is considered to be the degree of stretching of the ventricles at the end of filling phase, i.e. *end-diastolic volume* or *end-diastolic pressure* (length–tension relationship).

→ leading to

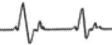

By increasing the filling of left ventricle during diastole → left ventricular force generation/systolic pressure can be increased up to optimal length/preload. Diastolic filling beyond optimal limits leads to decrease in systolic pressure (force/tension).

Afterload corresponds to the load against which the ventricle is to eject blood, i.e. it is correlated with the maximum systolic pressure of the left ventricle or the aortic pressure (force–velocity relationship). At constant preload, higher left ventricular systolic pressure can be achieved by increasing afterload (aortic pressure) up to certain limit.

When the afterload becomes so great that the left ventricle cannot increase its force (systolic pressure) further, the aortic valves fail to open. At this instant, though the force generated is maximum, the contraction is isometric, no external work is performed and velocity of shortening is zero. Force and velocity are inversely related and are dependent upon the intracellular concentration of free calcium ions. At constant velocity, force is equal to afterload, during shortening of the muscle. If the afterload is zero, the velocity of shortening is maximum.

→ leading to

5

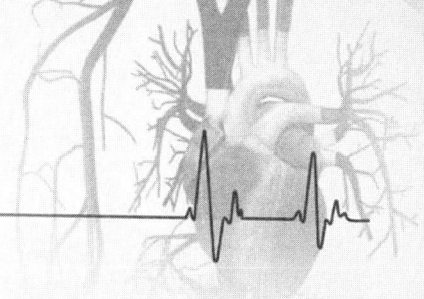

Electrocardiogram

NORMAL ELECTROCARDIOGRAM

Principle

As the cardiac impulse generated in the SA node passes through the heart, the electrical potentials not only spread through the heart, but also to the adjacent tissues and to the surface of the body, as body fluids are good volume conductors. The recording of these electrical potentials from the surface of the body is called *electrocardiogram* and the equipment is called *electrocardiograph*.

Lungs are filled with air and fluids of the other tissues surrounding the heart conduct electricity easily. When a portion of the ventricle becomes electronegative with respect to the remainder, current flows from depolarised area to the polarised area in large circuitous routes. For most of the time except for a short while, i.e. 1/100th second, the current flows in the direction from base to apex, with the depolarisation spreading from interventricular septum through endocardial surfaces of the ventricles, to apex of the heart. The last portions to be depolarised are the outer walls of the ventricles near the base of heart.

The monophasic action potential can be recorded with a microelectrode inserted into the single ventricular muscle fibre. The upsweep of action potential is caused by depolarisation of the ventricular muscle and the return of the potential to the baseline is due to repolarisation. No potential is recorded

21

when the ventricular muscle is either completely polarised or completely depolarised.

The normal electrocardiogram (Fig. 5.1) consists of a P wave due to atrial depolarisation, a QRS complex consisting of the Q wave, the R wave and the S wave, all due to ventricular depolarisation and the T wave due to ventricular repolarisation. The atrial repolarisation wave is undermined under the ventricular "*QRS*" complex. The electrical events in the cardiac cycle precede the mechanical events. The process of repolarisation in ventricular muscle occurs 0.25 to 0.35 seconds after depolarisation causing the T wave in the electrocardiogram.

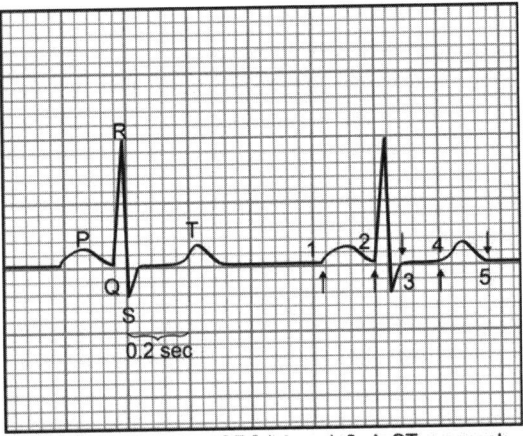

1–2: PR interval; 2–3: QRS interval; 3–4: ST segment;
3–5: ST interval; 2–5: QT interval

Fig. 5.1: Normal electrocardiogram

The depolarisation spreads through the muscle to initiate mechanical contraction. P wave occurs at the beginning of contraction of atria and QRS complex at the beginning of contraction of the ventricles. The ventricles remain contracted until the completion of repolarisation, i.e. the end of T wave. The atrial T wave occurs about 0.15 to 0.2 seconds after termination of the P wave.

The ventricular repolarisation wave is the T wave of the electrocardiogram. In some fibres of ventricular muscle, repolarisation starts 0.2 seconds after the beginning of

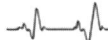

depolarisation wave (QRS complex). However, in some fibres it takes 0.35 seconds. Thus repolarisation extends to about 0.15 seconds.

METHODS OF RECORDING

Polarities and potentials of the electrical currents change very fast. The apparatus for recording electrocardiogram should be able to respond rapidly to the changes in potentials.

In the *pen type of recorder*, the pen, which is a thin tube connected at one end to an ink-well, and the other recording end to a powerful electromagnet system, directly writes on a moving sheet of paper. The electronic amplifiers connected to the electrocardiographic electrodes control the movement of the pen and the pen moves back and forth at high speed.

In the other system of recording, the recording stylus becomes hot by electrical current flowing through its tip and the paper turns black when exposed to heat.

Voltage and Time Calibration Lines

There are calibration lines on recording paper. In the pen type recorder, these lines are already there on the paper.

Horizontal Calibration Lines

These are voltage calibration lines. 10 small divisions in the upward or downward direction represent 1 mV. Positivity is indicated in the upward direction and negativity in the downward direction.

Vertical Calibration Lines

These are time calibration lines. Each inch, i.e. 2.5 cm, is equal to 1 second, which is broken into 5 segments by dark lines, the interval being 0.2 seconds. These intervals are further broken by thin lines into 5. Each of these represents 0.04 seconds.

VOLTAGES OF DIFFERENT WAVES AND INTERVALS

Normal Voltages

The potentials recorded are 3–4 mV, if electrodes are placed directly over the surface of the heart. The monophasic action

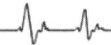

potential is 110 mV. The QRS wave, i.e. from the top of R wave to bottom of S wave is 1.0 –1.5 mV normally. Voltage of P wave is 0.1 to 0.3 mV. The T wave is 0.2 to 0.3 mV.

PR Interval

It is the time interval between the beginning of P wave to the beginning of QRS complex. It also denotes time interval between the beginning of contraction of atria to the beginning of contraction of ventricles and the time taken for conduction of impulse from atria to ventricles. Normal PQ or PR interval is 0.12 to 0.2 seconds (0.16 sec).

QRS Complex

It is the duration denoting ventricular depolarisation and atrial repolarisation. It is 0.08 to 0.1 seconds.

QT Interval

It is the time interval between the beginning of the Q wave to the end of T wave. The contraction of ventricles occurs during this time. It is 0.35–0.43 seconds.

ST Interval

It is QT minus QRS. It is about 0.32 seconds. It denotes ventricular repolarisation.

Heart Rate

Heart rate is the reciprocal of the time interval between two heart beats, i.e. the R-R interval. Therefore, if R-R interval is 0.83 seconds, heart rate is $1/0.83 \times 60$ which is equal to 72 beats per minute.

ELECTROCARDIOGRAPHIC LEADS

A lead consists of two wires and their electrodes, connecting the body with the electrocardiograph, making a complete circuit.

ECG is recorded by using an active or exploring electrode, connected to an indifferent electrode at zero potential (unipolar recording) or by using two active electrodes (bipolar recording).

The following is the classification of leads:
1. Bipolar limb leads
2. Unipolar augmented limb leads
3. Unipolar chest leads

There are three standard bipolar limb leads (Fig. 5.2A). The bipolar limb leads imply that the ECG is recorded from a pair of electrodes placed over the limbs.

Lead I : Negative terminal of electrocardiograph is connected to the right arm and positive terminal to the left arm.

Lead II : Negative terminal of electrocardiograph is connected to the right arm and positive terminal to left leg.

Lead III : Negative terminal of electrocardiograph is connected to the left arm and positive terminal to the left leg.

Einthoven's Law

It states that at any given instant, if the electrical potentials of any two of the three electrocardiographic bipolar limb leads are known, the third one can be determined mathematically from the first two by simply summing them (taking into consideration the positive and negative signs, i.e. algebraic sum).

If right arm is 0.3 mV negative with respect to average potential in the body, left arm is 0.4 mV positive and left leg is 1.2 mV positive, then:

Lead I : VL–VR = +0.4– (–0.3)=0.7 mV positive
Lead II : VF–VR = 1.2 –(–0.3) = 1.5 mV positive
Lead III : VF–VL = 1.2–(+0.4) = 0.8 mV positive

Thus the sum of the potentials recorded in lead I and III is equal to the potentials obtained in lead II.

Einthoven's Triangle

It is a diagrammatic means of illustrating that the two arms and the left leg form apices of an imaginary triangle surrounding the heart, with the heart in centre. The two arms electrically connect with the fluids around the heart at the two apices in the upper part of triangle. The lower apex of the triangle represents the point at which left leg connects with body fluids.

Augmented Unipolar Limb Leads (Fig. 5.2B)

In the augmented unipolar limb leads, two limbs are connected to the negative terminal of the electrocardiograph through electrical resistances. The third limb, at which the potentials are to be recorded, is connected to the positive terminal.

Lead aVR: Positive terminal on right arm

Lead aVL: Positive terminal on left arm

Lead aVF: Positive terminal on left leg

In the lead aVR, the P, QRS complex and the T wave are recorded as downward or negative deflections. This lead looks at the cavities of ventricles and the direction of depolarisation and repolarisation of atria and ventricles is away from exploring electrode.

In the leads aVL and aVF, the recordings are positive or biphasic.

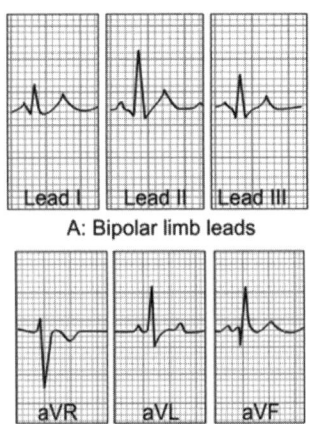

A: Bipolar limb leads

B: Augmented unipolar limb leads

Fig. 5.2A and B: Standard electrocardiographic limb leads

Chest Leads (Precordial Leads) (Fig. 5.3)

The active electrode is placed on the anterior surface of the chest, over the location of the heart, at the various designated locations and is connected to the positive terminal of the electrocardiograph. The negative electrode called the indifferent electrode, is connected through 5000 ohms electrical resistance to the right arm, left arm and left leg. Six standard chest leads are recorded, designated V_1, V_2, V_3, V_4, V_5 and V_6. The heart surfaces are close to the chest wall. Hence, each chest lead records the electrical potential of the cardiac musculature underneath the electrode. In leads V_1 and V_2 there is a small upward deflection as initially the ventricular depolarisation spreads from left to right across the septum. The chest electrode in these leads is nearer to the base of the heart than to the apex. Base of the heart is electronegative during most of the ventricular depolarisation process. The QRS recordings of the normal heart are mainly negative in leads V_1 and V_2 (large 'S' wave).

The QRS complexes in leads V_4, V_5 and V_6 are mainly positive. The chest electrodes in these leads are nearer to the apex of the heart and this area is electropositive during most of the depolarisation. A small 'Q' wave initially, followed by large R wave due to ventricular depolarisation moving towards exploring electrode and an 'S' wave due to depolarisation wave moving towards base of the ventricle are characteristic of these leads.

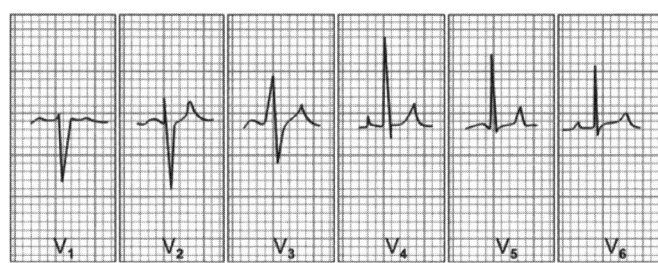

Fig. 5.3: Chest leads

Axis of limb leads

Each pair of electrodes (lead) is connected to the body on opposite sides of the heart. The direction from negative to positive electrode is called the *axis of the lead*. Lead I is horizontal and hence the axis is 0°. Lead II has an axis of +60° and lead III has an axis of +120°. The *hexagonal reference system* (Fig. 5.4) shows the directions of the axes of all the leads.

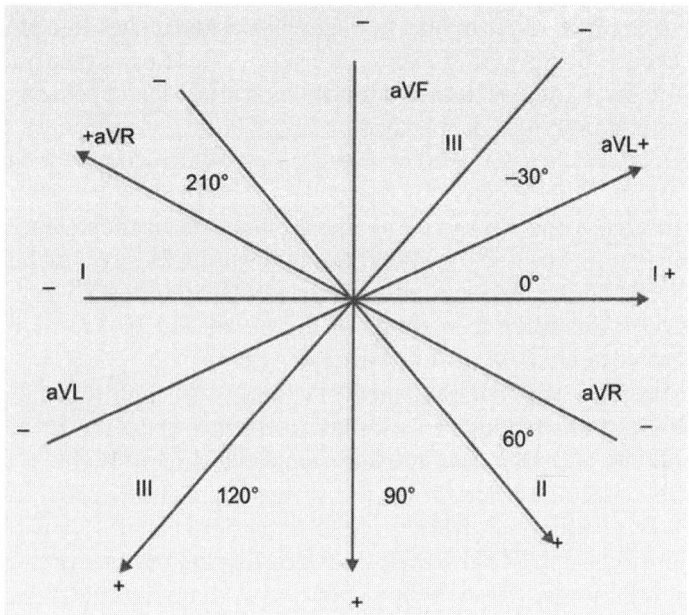

Fig. 5.4: Hexagonal reference system

DEFINITION OF VECTOR AND VECTORIAL ANALYSIS

A vector represents the changing potentials across the heart that occurs during cardiac cycle. The current flows in a particular direction in the cardiac cycle. Vector has a direction and magnitude. It is represented by an arrow, which points in the direction of electrical potential generated by the current flow, with the arrowhead in the positive direction. The length of the arrow is shown as proportional to the voltage of the potential.

Instantaneous Mean Vector

This vector represents the mean direction of current flow and the magnitude of the potentials generated by the heart at a particular instant. Initially, at the beginning of cardiac cycle, with the depolarisation of ventricular septum and parts of lateral endocardial walls, electrical current flows from inside to outside of the heart to the non-depolarised areas and also within the chambers from depolarised to polarised areas. Though some current flow occurs upwards, majority flows downward on the outside of the ventricles towards the apex. The summated vector at this particular instant is from the base to apex and is known as *instantaneous mean vector*.

Analysis of Vectors

The direction of the vector is represented in degrees and from zero reference point this rotates clockwise (downwards +90°, left to right 180° and upward –90° or 270°). If the instantaneous mean potentials in the ventricles during the depolarisation and the direction of the vector are known, projected vectors can be drawn to join the various lead axes of the standard bipolar limb leads and the magnitude and the direction of the potentials that would be recorded at that instant for the QRS complex in those leads can be obtained (Fig. 5.5).

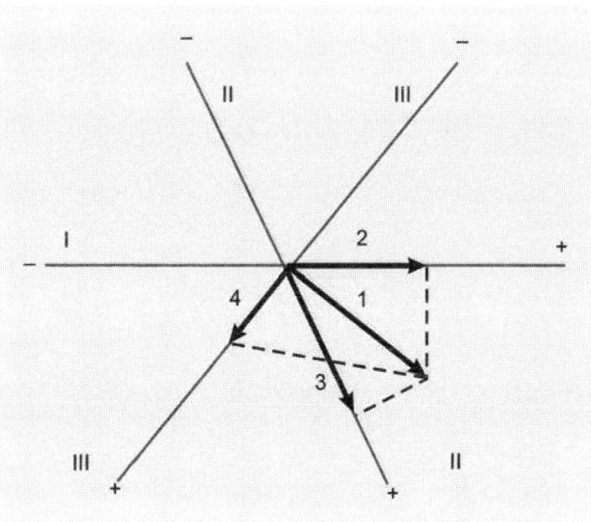

Fig. 5.5: Projected vectors 1. Instantaneous mean vector; 2, 3 and 4. Projected vectors for standard limb leads I, II and III respectively, all positive

Construction of Normal ECG (QRS Complex) from Various Instantaneous Mean Vectors

From the instantaneous mean vectors (having both magnitude and direction) that occur at successive intervals during depolarisation of the ventricles, the QRS complex can be constructed for each of the three standard bipolar limb leads, by drawing projected vectors. Positive vector in a lead results in positive deflection. Negative vector in a lead results in negative deflection.

First part of the ventricles to be depolarised is the left endocardial surface of the septum and then both endocardial surfaces. The depolarisation then spreads along both endocardial surfaces of the ventricles through the ventricular muscles to the outside of the heart.

Some times there is a Q wave due to initial depolarisation of the left side of the septum, creating a weak vector from left to right.

MEAN QRS VECTOR AND ELECTRICAL AXIS OF HEART (Fig. 5.6)

In normal heart, average direction of the vector of the heart during spread of the depolarisation wave through the ventricles, is from base to apex (Fig. 5.6). This preponderant direction of

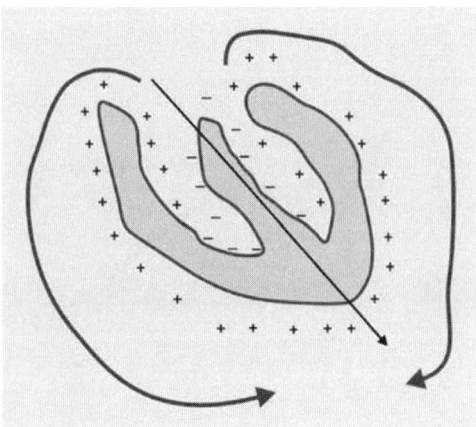

Fig. 5.6: Mean QRS vector. Mean QRS vector is depicted through the partially depolarised ventricles. It is +59°

the potential during depolarisation is called *mean QRS vector* or *mean electrical axis of ventricular QRS* and is +59°. During most of the ventricular depolarisation, the apex remains positive with respect to base.

Determination of Electrical Axis

The electrical axis of the heart or mean QRS vector can be known from the maximum potential and polarity of the recording of electrocardiogram in 2 or 3 standard bipolar limb leads (Fig. 5.7).

If any part of the recording is negative, this is subtracted from positive potential to know the net potential. Then these are plotted on the axes of the leads, with base of the potential at the point of intersection of the axes. If net potential is positive, it is

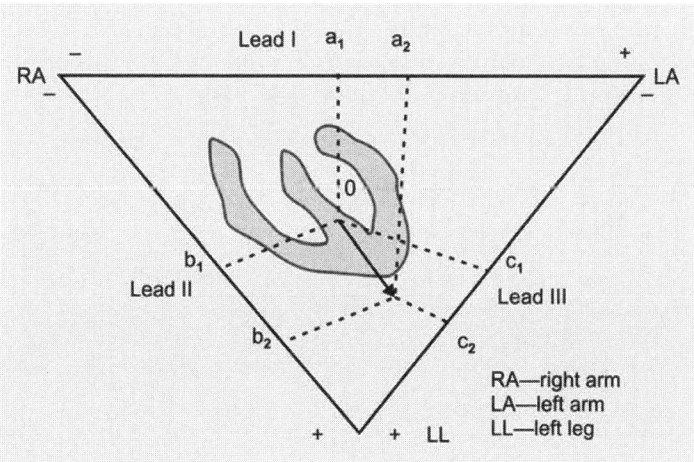

Fig. 5.7: Einthoven's triangle showing determination of mean QRS vector. Net potentials of all the three limb leads are shown here.

I. Perpendiculars drawn from the central points of sides of equilateral triangle (a_1, b_1, c_1), representing three limb leads, intersect at the centre of electrical activity (0)

II. From the height of R wave, the largest negative deflection is subtracted and plotted on each lead axis, from the mid-point of the side of the triangle (a_1–a_2; b_1–b_2; c_1–c_2)

III. An arrow is drawn from point '0' to the point of intersection of perpendiculars drawn from a_2, b_2 and c_2. This represents the mean QRS vector, its magnitude and its direction.

plotted in the positive direction along the lead axis. To determine the mean QRS vector, perpendiculars are drawn from the apices of 2 net potentials of leads I and III. The point of intersection represents the apex of the mean QRS vector and is joined to the point of intersection of the two lead axes.

VECTORCARDIOGRAM

As the impulse spreads, the current flow changes rapidly.

1. Vector changes in length as the voltages increase and decrease.
2. Vector changes its direction because the average direction of electrical potential of the heart changes.

Vectorcardiogram depicts changes in the voltages and direction of vectors at different instants during cardiac cycle. By joining the positive ends of instantaneous QRS vectors, the QRS vectorcardiogram is obtained (Fig. 5.8).

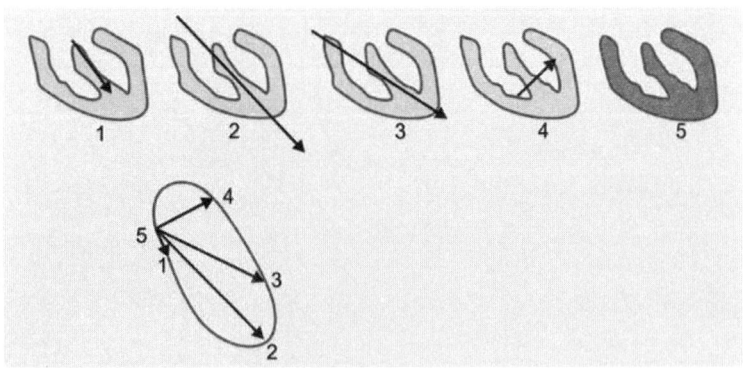

Fig. 5.8: QRS vectorcardiogram

Electrocardiogram during Repolarisation of Ventricles

The T wave: After the depolarisation of the ventricle, 0.15 seconds lapse, after which repolarisation starts. It is complete 0.35s after the onset of QRS complex. The septum and the endocardial area of the ventricles, which are first to depolarise, remain contracted for long time, their coronary flow is compromised and repolarise last.

The apical surfaces of the ventricles repolarise before the inner, basal surfaces and the positive end of the heart vector points downwards. Thus the vector during repolarisation points in a direction from base to apex, which is also the predominant direction during depolarisation. Hence, the T wave is positive in the 3 leads. The T wave is generated over about 0.15 seconds.

Electrocardiogram during Depolarisation of Atria

P wave: Depolarisation begins in SA node and spreads in all directions. The point of electronegativity is at the SA node and the direction of depolarisation and the vector remain the same throughout atrial depolarisation. The P wave is upright. Spread of depolarisation is much slower. SA node becomes depolarised long time before the depolarisation of other distal parts of atria. SA node area is repolarised first and hence the repolarisation vector is in opposite direction to that of depolarisation vector. The repolarisation occurs 0.15 seconds after P wave and is undermined under the QRS.

INTERPRETATION OF ECG

1. Cardiac rate and rhythm
2. Complete sequence
3. Voltage, duration and polarity of each wave
4. PR interval, QT interval, ST segment
5. Level of TP or ST segment in relation to baseline
6. Electrical axis of heart
7. Any abnormal wave

ABNORMALITIES

1. Abnormalities of rhythm
2. Conduction defects
3. Myocardial ischaemia and infarction
4. Ventricular hypertrophy
5. Abnormalities due to changes in serum electrolytes

Rhythm Abnormalities

Abnormalities in SA node or an abnormal focus of discharge in AV node, Purkinje fibres, atria or ventricles.

Sinus Arrhythmia

Characteristics
1. Some adults and most children have an increase in heart rate during inspiration and decrease during expiration.
2. Most evident during voluntary deep breathing or breath holding and is abolished during exercise.

Possible Mechanism
1. Negative intrathoracic pressure during inspiration → greater flow of blood into atria from veins → stretching of right atrium and SA node → increase in heart rate → Bainbridge reflex
2. Spill over of impulses from medullary respiratory centre to adjacent vasomotor centre.

Sinus Bradycardia

Characteristic
- Heart rate (RR interval): <60/minute.

Causes
1. Found in athletes
2. With increase in intracranial pressure
3. Hypothyroidism

Sinus Tachycardia

Characteristic
- Heart rate (RR interval) at rest: >90 beats per minute.

Causes
1. Emotional stress
2. Fever

→ leads to

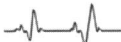

3. Exercise
4. Anaemia
5. Hyperthyroidism

Atrial Premature Beat or Extrasystole

Characteristics

1. P wave occurs early in heart cycle, PR interval is shortened (especially if the abnormal focus is near AV node), abnormal P wave, may be inverted.
2. The interval between the premature contraction and next normal contraction is prolonged, as the impulse generated from abnormal focus discharges SA node late during the premature beat and hence the sinus node discharges late for the next normal cycle. This interval is known as *compensatory pause*.
3. *Pulse deficit:* The stroke volume during the premature beat being less or absent, the pulse does not appear at the wrist. Hence there is a difference between the number of heart contractions and the pulse rate. This is known as *pulse deficit.*

Causes

1. Normal healthy people, smoking, lack of sleep, too much coffee intake, alcoholism
2. Ectopic foci due to:
    a. Areas of ischaemia
    b. Calcified plaques that press and cause irritable foci to develop in the myocardium
    c. Toxic irritation of the myocardium or excitatory and conductive system of heart by various drugs like nicotine or caffiene.

Atrial Paroxysmal Tachycardia

Abnormal focus generates impulses at a regular rate.

Characteristics

1. Inverted P wave, partially superimposed onto the normal T wave of preceding beat

2. Nodal tachycardia–aberrant rhythm in AV node
3. QRS is normal, P wave is missing

Cause

Both the tachycardias known as *supraventricular tachycardias* occur in young healthy people.

Atrial Flutter

Heart rate is 200 to 350/min.

Characteristics

1. Saw-tooth pattern of flutter waves due to atrial contractions
2. Accompanied with 2:1 or greater AV block

Cause

• Circus movement of the rhythm caused by irritable focus.

Atrial Fibrillation

Atria beat at the rate of 300–500/min and *"f"* waves can be diagnosed by electrocardiogram. No organized and effective atrial contraction is possible. Ripples traverse surface of the atria. Only some of the atrial impulses reach the ventricles and ventricular rate is irregular. QRS complexes are irregular (Fig. 5.9).

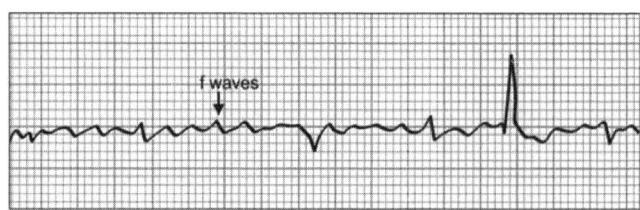

Fig. 5.9: Atrial fibrillation, lead V_1 showing fibrillatory waves (f waves)

Characteristics

1. Irregular atrial activity, chaotic rhythm
2. Fibrillatory (undulating) waves seen in V_1 and V_2
3. Variable RR interval

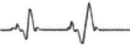

Causes

1. Infection
2. Fever
3. Hyperthyroidism
4. Metabolic or electrolyte abnormalities
5. Cardiomyopathy, myocardial infarction, valvular heart disease, hypertension, coronary artery disease, alcohol, sick sinus syndrome and pulmonary embolism

Ventricular Extrasystole

Abnormal focus in the ventricles discharges sporadically. During the relaxation period, cardiac muscle is in the relative refractory period. Strong electrical stimulus during this period leads to a contractile response. There is a compensatory pause, as the next natural impulse arrives during the refractory period of the heart and a normally expected contraction is missed (Fig. 5.10).

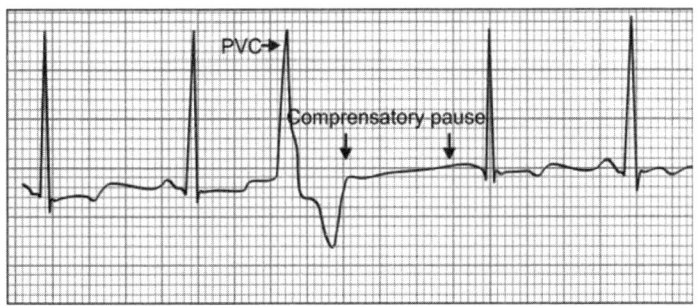

Fig. 5.10: Ventricular extrasystole (premature ventricular contraction, PVC)

Characteristics

1. An extrasystole manifests as a bizarre-shaped, prolonged QRS complex not preceded by a P wave.
2. The P wave is absent as it is buried under QRS.
3. The T wave is negative as the direction of repolarisation is not the same as that of depolarisation.
4. Normal impulse reaching the ventricles finds them in refractory period. Ventricles respond to next succeeding

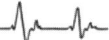
impulse from SA node. Hence, there is long compensatory pause.

5. It is not strong enough to produce pulse at the wrist.

Cause

An irritable ectopic focus in the ventricles discharges before the next impulse from the SA node.

Paroxysmal Ventricular Tachycardia

It can be supraventricular such as *paroxysmal nodal tachycardia* or *paroxysmal ventricular tachycardia.*

Characteristic

• *Torsade de pointes:* A form of ventricular tachycardia in which QRS morphology varies. It is seen as a number of ventricular premature beats, in quick succession to each other.

Cause

• Rapid ventricular depolarisation due to circus movement. The aberrant rhythm/irritable foci occur due to ischaemic damage of the ventricles.

This is a serious condition as ventricular fibrillation often follows.

Ventricular Fibrillation

Abnormal focus of impulse generation in the ventricles leads to ineffective disorganized contractions of the ventricles.

Characteristic

• Electrical activity of the heart is completely disorganized. Series of ineffective ventricular contractions look like *bag of worms*. Results in death within a few minutes.

Causes

Ventricular muscle fibres contract in irregular and ineffective way, due to multiple ectopic foci discharging at the same time

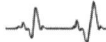

or circus movement (re-entry of the impulse) and continued propagation of the impulse in a long pathway, e.g.

1. Dilated hearts
2. Decreased conduction rate:
    a. Blockage in Purkinje system
    b. Ischaemia of ventricular muscle (myocardial infarction)
3. Repetitive electrical stimulation
4. When a person is electrocuted

Treatment

Defibrillator is used. High current of 110V, 60Hz is applied to the heart.

Wolff-Parkinson-White (WPW) Syndrome

Characteristics of the waveform

1. Short PR interval followed by delta wave
2. Prolonged QRS (>120 m sec)

Cause

Aberrant ventricular conduction due to accessory pathway

Symptoms

Asymptomatic or associated with tachycardia

Conduction Defects

Decrease in the efficiency of AV node, increase in AV delay result in different degrees of heart block.

SA Node Block

Whole heartbeat is lost. There is a pause when no atrial or ventricular contraction occurs. After an interval of less than 2 cardiac cycles, heart resumes normalcy. The condition is unmasked by exercise. It can be produced by vagal stimulation.

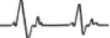

AV Block [AV Nodal Block or Block in the AV Bundle Fibres (Infranodal Block)]

Partial Heart Block

1st degree: PR interval >0.2 seconds

2nd degree heart block: 2:1 or 3:1 rhythm, i.e. 2 or 3 atrial beats followed by ventricular contraction

Wenckebach Phenomenon

PR intervals prolong gradually until a ventricular beat is dropped.

Complete Heart Block

Ventricles beat with slower independent rhythm, dictated by a portion of conducting tissue below the site of the block. If sudden complete heart block occurs, there is asystole, dizziness, loss of consciousness, convulsions and even death. This is known as *Stokes-Adams syndrome.*

Characteristics
1. The P and QRST complexes are normal but bear no relation to each other.
2. *AV nodal block:* Ventricular rate is 45/min. Infranodal block-rate 15/minute or so.
3. P waves are more in number than QRST.

Causes of AV Block
1. Extreme stimulation of vagus
2. Ischaemia due to coronary insufficiency
3. Compression due to calcification
4. Inflammation of AV node or bundle of His. Diphtheria or rheumatic myocarditis
5. Surgical corrections for interventricular septal defects
6. Septal infarction

Bundle Branch Block

When there is a block in one of the branches of bundle of His, the cardiac impulse cannot be propagated to the affected side normally, but the impulse can be conducted to the affected side through the ventricular syncytium. The duration of QRS complexes becomes more than 0.12 seconds. The electrical axis of the heart shifts accordingly.

Right Bundle Branch Block (Fig. 5.11)

Characteristics

1. Slurring of R wave with QRS ≥ 120 m sec in V_1 (rSR' pattern), V_2 and aVR, right axis deviation
2. R wave larger in amplitude than S wave in V_1 or V_2
3. Slurred S wave in V_5, V_6 and aVL
4. T wave is inverted in V_1 or V_2

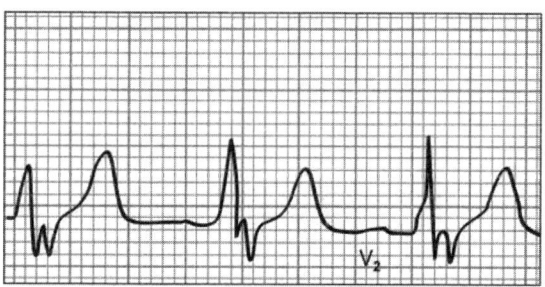

Lead V_2 showing prominent and broad R wave

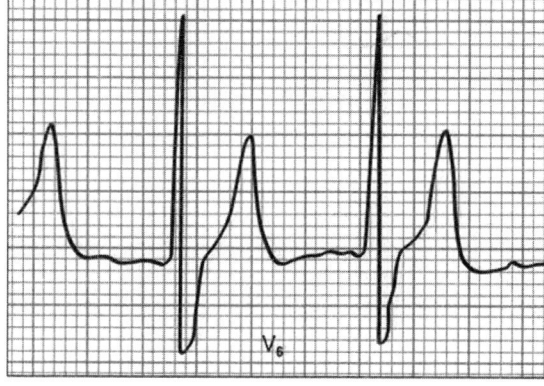

Lead V_6 showing broad S wave

Fig. 5.11: Right bundle branch block

Causes

1. Mechanical trauma to the right bundle (catheter)
2. Increased right ventricular pressure
3. Myocardial ischaemia or infarction (MI) of interventricular septum involving right branch of bundle of His.

Left Bundle Branch Block (Fig. 5.12)

Characteristics

1. Slurred broad R wave in V_4, V_5 and V_6 with QRS $\geq$ 120 m sec in all these leads and lead I
2. Poor R wave progression in V_1 to V_4
3. T wave is inverted in lead I, V_5 and V_6

Causes

1. Severe trauma to anterior or posterior fascicles
2. Myocardial ischaemia or infarction in the septal region involving left branch of bundle of His
3. May be associated with left ventricular hypertrophy/ dilatation
4. Fibrosis of conduction system (Lenegre's disease)

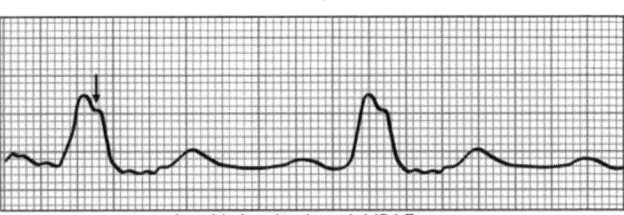

Lead I showing broad, bifid R wave

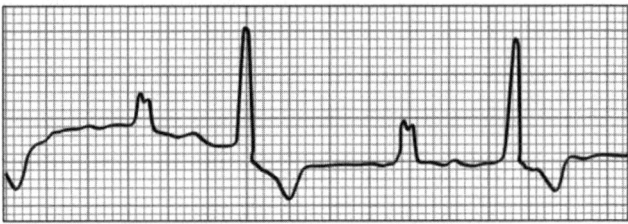

Lead V_6 showing broad R wave alternating with
premature ventricular contraction

Fig. 5.12: Left bundle branch block

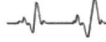

Right Axis Deviation

The normal axis of the heart varies from 20 to 100° (59° is mean electrical axis). When the axis of the heart shifts towards right, it is known as *right axis deviation*.

Causes

1. Can be normal in young people, athletes
   a. At the end of deep inspiration
   b. When a person stands up
   c. Tall, lean people
2. Lung disease, pulmonary embolism
3. Right ventricular hypertrophy due to:
   a. Congenital pulmonary valve stenosis
   b. Fallot's tetralogy
   c. Interventricular septal defect
4. Right bundle branch block

Symptoms

Symptoms consistent with lung disease or sharp pleuritic chest pain.

Left Axis Deviation

Characteristic

Marked left axis deviation, when the electrical axis is ≥ –30° or intense deviation when it is > –45°.

Causes

1. Electrical axis of heart normally varies from 20° to 100°:
   a. At the end of deep expiration
   b. When a person lies down, due to pressing of abdominal contents against diaphragm
   c. In obese people
2. Left ventricular hypertrophy:
   a. Greater quantity of muscle, greater time for the impulse to travel
   b. Excess generation of potential on left side
3. Left anterior fascicular block or hemiblock

4. Hypertension
5. Inferior myocardial infarction

Ventricular Hypertrophy

Prolonged work by any muscle leads to adaptive hypertrophy. Adaptive hypertrophy to volume or pressure load occurs in the ventricles.

Right Ventricular Hypertrophy

Right ventricle may be overloaded by increase in pulmonary vascular resistance or left to right shunt.

Characteristics

1. Increase in ventricular mass leads to increased magnitude of currents generated during the spread of cardiac impulse. Increased size means increase in the time taken by the cardiac impulse to spread through the hypertrophied ventricle. There may be prolongation of QRS complex but may not be so marked. As the hypertrophied ventricle takes longer time and remains electropositive, there is stronger electric current flow from normal to hypertrophied ventricle and there is corresponding right axis deviation.
2. R wave is greater than 'S' in V_1 and V_2.

Causes

1. Chronic obstructive pulmonary disease
2. Primary and secondary pulmonary hypertension
3. Pulmonary embolus and congenital heart disease

Left Ventricular Hypertrophy (Fig. 5.13)

Characteristics

1. Large S wave in V_1 and V_2.
2. R wave >15 mm in any limb lead, V_5 and V_6
3. Left axis deviation
4. *ST depression:* If present, indicates hypertension, diastolic and systolic left ventricular dysfunction, congestive heart failure, stroke and death of cardiac tissue

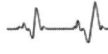

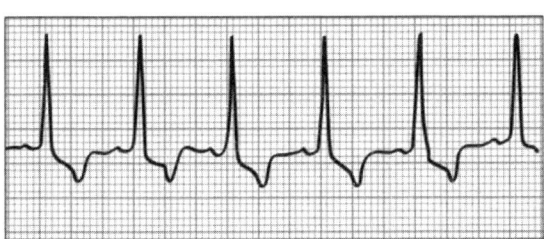

Fig. 5.13: Left ventricular hypertrophy with left ventricular strain, lead V_6 showing depressed ST segment

Causes

1. Hypertension
2. Aortic stenosis, aortic valve regurgitation, congenital heart disease

Left Atrial Enlargement: P mitrale

Characteristic

• Broad, notched P waves in lead II, aVF (>2.5 mm wide)

Causes

1. Mitral regurgitation
2. Congestive heart failure

Right Atrial Enlargement (P-pulmonale)

There are 2 humps in P wave (right atrial component – appears first)

• Tall, peaked P waves (>2.5 mm height)

Causes

Vertical axis due to:
1. Lung disease
2. Pulmonary embolus/hypertension

QT Prolongation

Characteristic

• When QT is >50 per cent of RR interval, QT prolongation occurs.

Causes

1. Associated with premature ventricular contraction, ventricular tachycardia and fibrillation
2. Hypocalcaemia, hypokalaemia and other electrolyte/metabolic abnormalities
3. Cardiac disease, myocardial infarction
4. Antiarrhythmic drugs

Myocardial Ischaemia

Maintenance of normal resting membrane potential (RMP) requires metabolic activity, normal blood supply providing oxygen and nutrients and removal of metabolic end products. Decrease in blood supply can abolish RMP, though it may not be severe enough to cause death of the tissue. Hence the ischaemic zone is electronegative as compared to healthy myocardium in both myocardial ischaemia and myocardial infarction, from which there is a flow of current from the injured region to the healthy myocardium. This is known as *current of injury*. The configuration of ECG is altered.

Characteristics

Current of Injury: J Point: The point of return of the QRS to the zero reference level, or the point at which the entire ventricular muscle is depolarised (including the healthy and damaged) and there is no current flow, is known as *J point*.

1. Current of injury is abolished when whole of both the ventricles are depolarised because the injured zone becomes electrically similar to the healthy zone.
2. During TP interval, the current of injury is unadulterated as there is no interacting current.

For Diagnosis of Ischaemia or Infarction: The point where QRS ends, i.e. point where both ventricles are depolarised and there is no current flow is noted and this point is the J point. A horizontal line is drawn through this point. This indicates the level on the ECG where there is no current flow and is the true isoelectric line. The level of TP segment in relation to the isoelectric line is observed. Its direction (positive or negative) and magnitude may be noted in any two leads.

The direction in which current of injury points is from negative to positive region of heart, represented as an arrow from injured to healthy region of the heart. Thus, the positive electrode of a particular lead placed near to the healthy myocardium records positive deflection. The location of the infarct can be found out through specific leads. For example, the ECG can be recorded from a chest lead like V_2 (anterior lead). If there is positive current of injury in V_2, it suggests posterior infarct and if negative, anterior infarct.

1. For specific sites of infarction, the abnormalities appear in specific leads (Fig. 5.14):

   Anterior infarction—Leads I and V_1 to V_5
   Inferior infarction—Leads II, III , aVF, V_1 and V_2
   Lateral infarction—Leads I, aVL, V_5 and V_6
2. Q wave changes like prominences may persist.
3. *T wave inversion:* When the ventricular muscle takes longer time for depolarisation, then the polarity of the

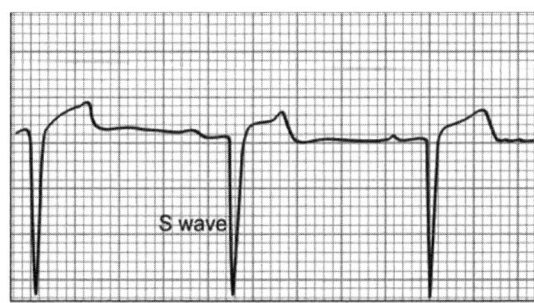

QS pattern in lead V_2, anterior wall myocardial infarction

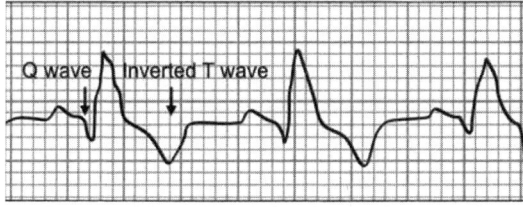

Q wave, inverted T wave in lead III, inferoposterior myocardial infarction

Fig. 5.14: Myocardial infarction

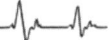

repolarisation wave changes and may result in inverted T wave.

Causes

1. Decrease in coronary blood flow due to atherosclerosis—coronary insufficiency.
2. Thrombosis, embolism or spasm of the artery supplying the myocardium, if severe enough leads to myocardial infarction and death of myocardium.

Anterior Myocardial Infarction

Characteristics

1. *Q waves*: Should be 40 milliseconds in duration, at least 25 per cent of the amplitude of the following R wave and should occur in any 2 of the anterior leads, i.e. V_2, V_3 and V_4. All the characteristics should be present for the Q waves to be diagnostic. QS complexes are seen in these leads.
2. ST elevation if recorded in the same lead suggests recent myocardial infarction.

Cause

- Lesion/thrombosis in the left anterior descending coronary artery

Septal Infarction

Characteristic

- *Q waves:* All above abnormal features of Q waves in V_1 and V_2. QS pattern seen in V_1 and V_2.

Causes

1. Septal infarct
2. Can occur due to faulty placement of electrodes
3. Anatomical changes like vertical axis of the heart due to lung causes, left ventricular hypertrophy or conduction defects can produce similar QS pattern.

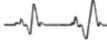

Inferior Infarction

Characteristic

- *Q waves:* All above abnormal features of Q waves in 2 of the inferior leads, i.e. leads II, III and aVF.

Cause

- Lesion/thrombus in right coronary artery and/or left circumflex artery.

Changes in Serum Electrolytes

The resting membrane potential is due to intracellular and extracellular electrolyte concentration differences and is responsible for the electrical activity of all excitable tissues of the body.

Hyponatraemia

Results in decrease in voltage in ECG.

Hyperkalaemia

1. Peaked, high voltage T waves
2. Slurred and greatly prolonged QRS complex
3. Stopping of atrial contraction, ventricular fibrillation

Hypokalaemia

1. Prolongation of PR interval
2. Prominent U wave with inverted T wave

Hypercalcaemia

Hypercalcaemia producing significant changes in ECG is rarely seen clinically.

Hypocalcaemia

Causes prolongation of ST segment and increase in QT interval.

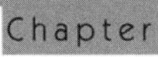

6

Laws Governing Circulation

The flow of blood in the straight blood vessels is streamline (laminar). Blood vessels are not rigid tubes. Blood is not a perfect fluid but an interface of cells and liquid plasma. However, the physical principles applied to rigid tubes and ideal fluids are some times applied for the purpose of understanding the flow dynamics.

Blood, like water or any fluid flows from high pressure areas to low pressure areas. Certain times, under contrary situations, momentum transiently sustains the flow. The relationship between mean flow, mean pressure and resistance can be compared to the relationship between current, electromotive force and resistance in an electrical circuit. This is expressed by Ohm's law.

OHM'S LAW

$$\text{Current (I)} = \frac{\text{Electromotive force (E)}}{\text{Resistance (R)}}$$

$$\text{Flow (F)} = \frac{\text{Pressure (P)}}{\text{Resistance (R)}}$$

$$\text{Or Resistance (R)} = \frac{\text{Pressure (P)}}{\text{Flow (F)}}$$

Units for resistance are dyne.s/cm^5 or R units.

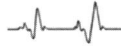

$$1 \text{ R unit} = \frac{100 \text{ mmHg}}{100 \text{ ml/sec}}$$

The pressure is actually pressure difference or effective perfusion pressure.

Effective perfusion pressure = Mean pressure (mean intra-luminal) at the arterial end—mean pressure at the venous end.

POISEUILLE-HAGEN FORMULA OR POISEUILLE'S LAW

$$\text{Flow (F)} = \left(P_A - P_B\right) \times \frac{\pi}{8} \times \frac{1}{\eta} \times \frac{r^4}{L}$$

$P_A - P_B$ = Pressure difference between the two ends of the tube
η = viscosity; r = radius of the tube; L = length of the tube

As flow is equal to pressure difference divided by resistance (R),

$$R = \frac{8\eta L}{\pi r^4}$$

Flow varies as 4th power of radius. Hence this is also known as 4th power law. Small changes in the calibre of arterioles, thus have profound effects on systemic arterial pressure.

VELOCITY AND FLOW

Velocity of flow in a system of tubes is defined as displacement per unit time (cm/s) and flow as volume per unit time (cm^3/s).

Velocity (V) is α Flow (F)

VELOCITY AND CROSS-SECTIONAL AREA

As the cross-sectional area increases, velocity of flow decreases. Velocity in the aorta is the greatest and it is the least in the capillaries.

V α 1/A

V = F/A or F = VA,

F = Flow; V = Velocity; A = Area

Thus if flow stays constant, velocity increases in proportion to any decrease in the area. The average velocity of fluid movement, at any point in a system of tubes in parallel, is inversely proportionate to the total cross-sectional area at that point. The velocity of blood flow is highest in the aorta, declining gradually in the smaller vessels. It is lowest in the capillaries, which, have the total cross-sectional area 1000 times that of the aorta. Average velocity of blood flow again increases as the blood enters veins and is high in the vena cava.

FLOW CHARACTERISTICS

Flow of Blood

Flow of blood is streamline or laminar. Laminar flow is silent. Turbulent flow creates sounds. Velocity of blood flow is greatest in the centre of the stream. Thus the profile of blood flow is said to be parabolic, with the velocity of the central lamina (sheet) being highest, the adjacent layers having lower velocities and the layer of blood in contact with the vessel wall having the lowest velocity. When the velocity of blood flow exceeds critical velocity, laminar flow becomes turbulent.

Reynold's Number

The probability of turbulence is directly related to the diameter of the vessel (D, in cm), velocity of flow (V, in cm/second), density of fluid (ρ) and inversely to the viscosity of the fluid (η, in poises). This probability is given by Reynold's number (Re).

$$\text{Re} = \frac{\rho D V}{\eta}, \text{ When R >2000, turbulence is present.}$$

Turbulent Flow Creates Eddy Currents

Turbulent flow is normally present:
1. In the ascending aorta, at the peak of systolic ejection
2. While measuring blood pressure, the pressure in the sphygmomanometer cuff is raised temporarily, to a value above estimated systolic pressure, thus producing artificial constriction. Flow is occluded in the brachial artery and sounds of "Korotkoff" are produced due to eddie currents.

Pathologically

1. In anaemia as viscosity is decreased.
2. Over arteries constricted by atherosclerotic plaques.

VISCOSITY AND RESISTANCE

Resistance to Blood Flow

It is determined by:

1. Radius of the blood vessels
2. Viscosity of blood

Viscosity of Blood

It depends on:

1. Viscosity of plasma
2. Haematocrit, i.e. percentage of the volume of blood occupied by red blood cells.

In small vessels (arterioles, capillaries and venules) less than 100 mm in diameter, the nature of flow is different. Hence, the effect of change in haematocrit has much less influence in changing viscosity as compared to large bore vessels. The overall effect of change in haematocrit on viscosity is less, until and unless the haematocrit changes drastically as in polycythaemia (10 times the viscosity of water).

The viscosity of plasma is 1.5 times that of water and the viscosity of whole blood is 3 times that of water.

Viscosity is also affected by plasma proteins and the resistance of cells to deformation, e.g.

1. ↑ immunoglobulins in plasma
2. Hereditary spherocytosis.

Conductance and Resistance

- Conductance = 1/resistance
- Conductance is a measure of blood flow through a vessel for a given pressure difference
- It can be expressed in mL or L/sec/mmHg
- Conductance α diameter^4

Critical Closing Pressure

In small vessels, when the pressure is reduced, there is no flow at a point of time, even when the pressure is not zero. Thus, it takes some pressure to force blood through the small, thin and delicate vessels, as these vessels remain in a collapsed state, due to pressure exerted on them by surrounding tissue fluid.

Law of Laplace

This law states that the tension (T) in the wall of a cylinder is equal to the product of transmural pressure (P) times the radius (r), divided by the wall thickness (w), i.e.

$$T = Pr/w.$$

The transmural pressure (pressure inside the capillary–pressure acting on the capillary from outside) in a thin-walled capillary (synonymous with cylinder here) is equal to pressure inside capillary, as the pressure acting outside (tissue pressure) is negligible. The wall thickness can also be ignored as the capillaries are thin walled.

Hence $P = T\left(\dfrac{1}{r_1} + \dfrac{1}{r_2}\right)$, where r_1 and r_2 are two principal radii of curvature

As $r_1 = r_2$ in a sphere, $P = \left(\dfrac{2T}{r}\right)$

However, in the blood vessel , one radius being infinite,

$$P = \left(\frac{T}{r}\right)$$

Hence, the tension required in the capillary wall to balance the distending pressure is very small. Thus fragile structures like capillaries having small radius, do not rupture due to operation of law of Laplace.

On the other hand, there is a disadvantage faced by dilated hearts due to operation of this law. The radius of the dilated cardiac chamber is increased and hence greater tension has to develop in the myocardium to produce a given pressure. Thus the dilated heart has to perform more work.

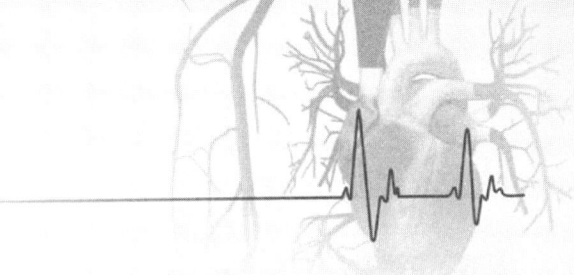

7

Cardiac Cycle

DEFINITION

All the events occurring in the heart from beginning of one heartbeat to the beginning of the next heartbeat are called *cardiac cycle*.

ATRIAL EVENTS

Atrial Systole

It is a period of atrial contraction. It immediately follows "P" wave of the electrocardiogram. It lasts for 0.1 seconds and causes "a" wave in the atrial pressure curve and jugular venous pulse.

Atrial contraction accounts for 20 per cent filling of ventricles and rest of the 80 per cent of the blood continuously flows from great veins through atria into ventricles. During the atrial systole, a fourth heart sound can be recorded by phonocardiogram, due to inrush of blood into the already filled ventricles. This is also known as *atrial heart sound*. As the heart has the capacity to pump 3–4 times the quantity of blood required by the body at rest, atrial failure is not noticed till a person exercises.

Atrial Diastole

Period of atrial relaxation. Lasts for 0.7 seconds.

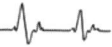
PRESSURE CHANGES IN ATRIA

a Wave

Increase in atrial pressure caused by atrial contraction. During atrial systole, right atrial pressure rises to 4–6 mmHg and left atrial pressure rises to 7–8 mmHg.

c Wave

It occurs when ventricles begin to contract. It is due to:
1. At the onset of ventricular contraction, there is slight backflow of blood into the atria.
2. Bulging of AV valves backward into the atria, due to increased pressure in the ventricles.

v Wave

Rise in atrial pressure due to slow flow of blood from the veins into the atria, while the ventricles are contracting and AV valves are closed. With the opening of the AV valves, blood flows rapidly into the ventricles and the "v" wave disappears.

VENTRICULAR EVENTS

Ventricular contraction starts after the wave of ventricular depolarisation in the ECG, the QRS wave. Ventricular systole lasts for 0.3 seconds approximately and ventricular diastole lasts for 0.5 seconds.

PERIOD OF ISOVOLUMIC CONTRACTION OR ISOMETRIC CONTRACTION

Immediately after ventricular filling, the ventricular pressure rises abruptly and the AV valves close, causing Ist heart sound. Ventricles start contracting and build up pressure for 0.02–0.03 seconds, so as to push the semilunar (aortic and pulmonary) valves open. During this period tension in the ventricular muscle is increasing but no shortening occurs (isometric—same length). Ventricles contract as closed chambers, with all the valves closed.

PERIOD OF EJECTION (0.22 s)

When left ventricular pressure rises above 80 mmHg and right ventricular pressure above 8 mmHg, the semilunar valves are pushed open.

• *Period of rapid ejection*: 1/3rd of the ejection phase; 70 per cent of the blood is ejected out.

• *Period of slow ejection*: 2/3rd of ejection phase; 30 per cent of the blood is ejected out.

As left ventricular pressure increases above the aortic pressure (80 mmHg), the aortic valve opens, blood starts flowing out of the left ventricle into the aorta and peak systolic pressure of 120 mmHg is reached in the left ventricle. However, during the later part of the ventricular systole, though the left ventricular pressure falls (as the blood is moving) below the aortic pressure (which is 120 mmHg), still blood keeps moving due to the built up momentum. This phase is known as *protodiastole* and lasts for 0.04 seconds. As the kinetic energy of the momentum is converted into pressure in the aorta, the aortic valve snaps shut (closes) causing the second heart sound.

THE AORTIC PRESSURE CURVE

As there is a short period of back flow of blood, followed by sudden cessation of back flow due to closure of aortic valves, incisura in the aortic pressure curve occurs. After the closure of aortic valves, elastic recoil of aorta maintains blood flow through the vessels to the entire body. As blood flows through the peripheral vessels, the aortic pressure drops to the diastolic value of 80 mmHg. The pressure in the pulmonary artery is 1/6th of the aorta.

PERIOD OF ISOVOLUMIC (ISOMETRIC) RELAXATION

At the end of systole, ventricular relaxation begins abruptly and ventricles relax as closed chambers for 0.03–0.06 seconds. Intraventricular pressures fall to low diastolic values below the intra-atrial pressure (as the atria were getting filled with blood returning from great veins) and the AV valves open. Opening of the valves does not produce sound, as this is a slow developing process.

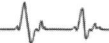

FILLING OF THE VENTRICLES

While the ventricles are contracting with AV valves closed, large amount of blood is collecting in the atria, causing "*v*" wave in the atrial pressure curve. As soon as ventricular systole is over and the ventricular pressures fall to low diastolic values, the atria push open the AV valves and blood flows rapidly into the ventricles. Ventricular filling is divided into three phases:

1. **Period of rapid filling (0.11 sec):** Rapid inflow of blood occurs during the first third of diastole.

2. **Diastasis (0.19 sec):** During the middle third of the diastole, only a small amount of blood flows into the ventricles, directly from the veins through the atria. At the beginning of the middle third of diastole, a rumbling third heart sound is recorded with the help of phonocardiogram.

   Possible explanation given: Oscillation of blood back and forth between the walls of ventricles, initiated by inrushing blood from atria.

   Rapid filling phase and diastasis account for 80 per cent (first 2/3rds) filling of the ventricles.

3. **Atrial systole (0.1 sec):** Rest of the 20 per cent of the filling of ventricles is due to contraction of the atria. Now as the intraventricular pressure exceeds the intra-atrial pressure, the AV valves close and the cycle repeats.

EJECTION FRACTION

It is an index of the contractile state of the myocardium. It is the ratio of the volume of blood ejected from the left ventricle per beat (stroke volume), to the volume of blood in the left ventricle at the end of diastole (end-diastolic volume). This is widely used as a clinical index. It is about 60 per cent.

The slope of the ascending limb of the ventricular pressure curve also indicates maximal rate of force development by the ventricle, which again is an index of contractility.

CONTRACTILITY

Contractility is defined as the change in peak isometric force (isovolumic pressure) at a given initial fibre length (end-diastolic volume).

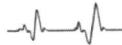

WORK OUTPUT OF THE HEART

There are two types of work output by the heart.

Stroke Work Output

The amount of energy that the heart converts to work, while pumping blood into arteries during each heartbeat, is known as *stroke work output.*

Minute Work Output

This is total amount of energy converted to work by the heart in one minute. This is equal to stroke work output times the heart rate per minute.

VOLUME PRESSURE WORK OR EXTERNAL WORK

Work performed by the left ventricle, to raise the pressure of blood during each heartbeat is known as external work. This work is performed by the left ventricle to move the blood from low pressure veins to the high pressure arteries. The work output of the right ventricle is 1/6th of left ventricle.

Left ventricular external work output = Stroke volume × (left ventricular mean ejection pressure – left ventricular mean input pressure during diastolic filling).

When pressure is in dynes/sq cm and stroke volume is in ml, the work output is in Ergs. Right ventricular external work output is about 1/6th the work output of left ventricle.

KINETIC ENERGY OF BLOOD FLOW COMPONENT

Minor proportion of the energy is used to accelerate the blood to its velocity of ejection through the aortic and pulmonary valves.

The additional work output of each ventricle, required to create kinetic energy of blood flow, is proportional to the mass of blood ejected times the square of velocity of ejection.

$$\text{Kinetic energy} = \frac{mV^2}{2}$$

When mass is expressed in grams of blood ejected and the velocity in centimeters per second, the work output is in Ergs. Normally the work output of the left ventricle, required to create kinetic energy of blood flow is 1 per cent of total work output and hence ignored in total calculation.

GRAPHICAL ANALYSIS OF VENTRICULAR PUMPING

Systolic Pressure Curve

The maximum pressure achieved during ventricular contraction, at each volume of filling of left ventricle (end-diastolic volume, EDV), can be determined by preventing any outflow of blood from left ventricle. This is maximum systolic pressure and can be plotted at each EDV. The systolic pressure increases as the EDV increases, but reaches peak value at an EDV of 150–170 ml. As the EDV increases further, systolic pressure actually decreases, because the actin and myosin filaments are pulled apart.

Diastolic Pressure Curve

Diastolic pressure is determined immediately before left ventricular contraction occurs, at a particular volume of filling. This is end-diastolic pressure (EDP) of the left ventricle. The heart is filled with progressively greater quantities of blood and the diastolic pressure (end-diastolic pressure, EDP) is measured immediately before the contraction of the left ventricle at each volume of filling (EDV). The end-diastolic pressure is plotted against end-diastolic volume.

When the EDV increases more than 150 ml, the diastolic pressure increases rapidly as the fibrous tissue of the heart hinders any further stretch and the pericardium is stretched nearly to its maximum. Also, as per definition of Starling's law of heart, the heart muscle (myocardium as a whole) has already been stretched beyond physiological limits.

The Volume Pressure Diagram (for the Left Ventricle)

It is divided into 4 phases:
  I. *Period of filling:* From end-systolic volume (ESV) of 45 ml, the ventricular volume increases to 115 ml (EDV). The end-diastolic pressure increases from 0 to 5 mmHg.

II. *Period of isovolumic contraction:* Volume does not change, pressure inside the ventricle increases above 80 mmHg, i.e. above the diastolic pressure in the aorta.

III. *Period of ejection:* The aortic valve opens at the beginning of this phase. Systolic pressure rises to higher values of 120 mmHg. The volume of ventricle decreases because blood flows out of aortic valve.

IV. *Period of isovolumic relaxation:* At the end of period of ejection, the aortic valve closes, ventricular pressure falls back to the diastolic pressure level. The ventricle returns to the starting point of 45 ml and 0 mmHg pressure.

ENERGY REQUIRED FOR CARDIAC CONTRACTION

Chemical energy is required for cardiac contraction. The heart requires oxygen for the work. Chemical energy is obtained by oxidative metabolism of fatty acids and other nutrients. Rate of oxygen consumption is proportional to the work output.

Efficiency of Cardiac Contraction

During heart muscle contraction, most of the chemical energy is converted to heat and a smaller portion into work output. Ratio of work output to total chemical energy expenditure is called the *efficiency of cardiac contraction* or *efficiency of the heart*. Maximum efficiency of normal heart is 20–25 per cent.

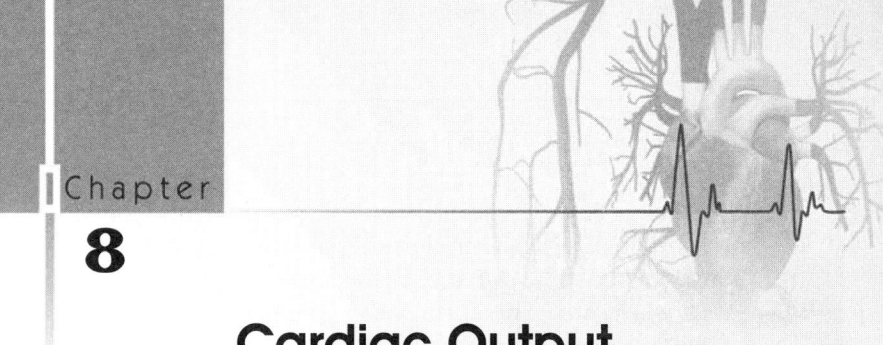

8

Cardiac Output

DEFINITIONS

Cardiac output is the quantity of blood pumped by the heart into the aorta, each minute. It is same as the amount of blood that flows through circulation and is responsible for transporting substances to and from the tissues. Venous return is the quantity of blood flowing from the veins into the right atrium each minute.

Cardiac output (CO) = Heart rate (HR) × Stroke volume (SV)

Stroke volume (SV) = End-diastolic volume (EDV) – End-systolic volume (ESV)

Normal resting cardiac output is 5 to 5. 6 liters/min.

STROKE VOLUME

The amount of blood pumped out of each ventricle per beat is known as the stroke volume and is 70–80 ml, with the 2 ventricular pumps working in series.

CARDIAC INDEX

The output per minute, per square metre of body surface area, is known as *cardiac index*. It averages 3. 1 to 3. 2 L/min/sq m.

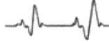

END-DIASTOLIC VOLUME (EDV), END-DIASTOLIC PRESSURE (EDP), END-SYSTOLIC VOLUME (ESV) AND STROKE VOLUME OUTPUT

EDV: Filling of the ventricles increases the volume of each ventricle to 110–120 ml. This volume is known as *end-diastolic volume*.

EDP: The pressure at the end of diastole is called *end-diastolic pressure*. As the walls of the ventricles are stretched and elastic structures in their walls tend to recoil, pressure develops in the ventricles.

Both EDV and EDP are indicators of preload, which is the volume load in the ventricles prior to contraction. During the systole, i.e. the contraction phase of the ventricles, the pump cycle muscles forming the chambers are active, i.e. excitation–contraction coupling occurs, muscle cells develop force → wall tension increases → increase in intraventricular pressure occurs! the aortic valve opens (left ventricular pressure exceeds the aortic pressure) → circumferential shortening, i. e. squeezing down on the volume of blood occurs in the left ventricle leading to ejection.

ESV: The ventricles do not completely empty and the residual volume is known as *end-systolic volume* (ESV). This is about 40–50 ml.

$$SV = EDV - ESV$$

NORMAL VARIABLES OF CARDIAC OUTPUT

Increases

1. Age (the cardiac index increases up to 10 years of age and then starts declining)
2. Level of activity, anxiety, excitement
3. High environmental temperature
4. Body metabolism, pregnancy
5. Exercise, epinephrine
6. Size of the body

Decreases

1. In women 10 to 20 per cent less, decreases in old age
2. In sitting or standing, from lying position

→ leading to

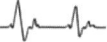

No change

Sleep, moderate changes in environmental temperature

CELLULAR MECHANICS AND CORRELATES OF CARDIAC FUNCTION

The number of cycling cross-bridges determines the cardiac function at the cellular level. This is regulated by:
1. Contractility or the level of Ca^{2+} activation
2. The sarcomere length
3. The afterload (velocity of shortening)

REGULATION (FACTORS CONTROLLING) OF CARDIAC OUTPUT

Primary Control

Cardiac output (CO) is equal to the product of heart rate and stroke volume. Factors affecting heart rate, stroke volume (EDV-ESV) and aortic pressure change the cardiac output.

Stroke Volume Depends On

EDV: End-diastolic volume represents the degree of filling of the ventricles and hence the initial length of the myocardium. As per Frank-Starling law of the heart, increase in the stretching of the myocardium leads to increased degree of contraction by the ventricles. At the cellular level, the increase in tension generated is due to increase in the number of cycling cross-bridges.

The left ventricular pressure increases and the heart functions as better pump. However, there is a limit to the extent to which the heart can be stretched.

Increases in end-diastolic volume (i.e. preload, degree of stretching) bring about increase in stroke volume. This is known as *length tension relationship or heterometric regulation.*

ESV: Decrease in end-systolic volume (degree of shortening, contractility) results in increase in stroke volume at constant EDV. Contractility is defined as the extent of shortening against afterload. It is primarily controlled by extrinsic factors and is known as *homometric regulation.*

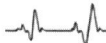

Afterload

Aortic pressure or arterial pressure is defined as afterload. It is dependent on peripheral resistance. This is also known as *force velocity relationship.*

Heart Rate

The extrinsic cardiac innervation is by sympathetic and parasympathetic nerves. Sympathetic stimulation increases the heart rate and parasympathetic stimulation decreases the heart rate.

Secondary Control

- *Renin-angiotensin system: System signal (juxtaglomerular cells):*
    i. Decreased mean arterial pressure (MAP)
    ii. Decreased pulse pressure in afferent arteriole
    iii. Reduction in plasma sodium
- *Atrial receptors/ADH (vasopressin)/ANF:*
    i. A receptors (pressure sensitive)
    ii. B receptors (volume sensitive)

HETEROMETRIC REGULATION (Fig. 8.1)

Frank and Starling, two great physiologists stated the *Frank-Starling mechanism of the heart* or *Frank-Starling law of the heart.* The intrinsic ability of the heart to adapt to changing volumes of inflowing blood (i. e. venous return, which is the sum of all the local blood flows) returning to right atrium, is called the

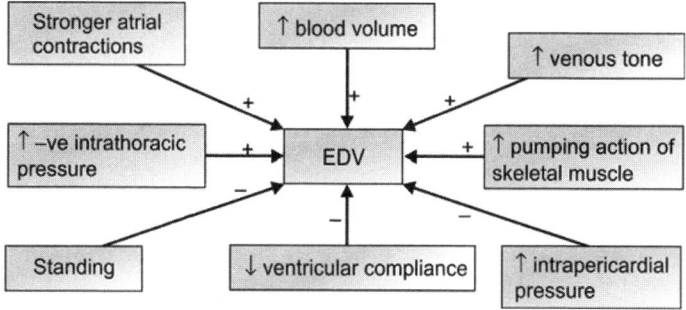

Fig. 8.1: Factors affecting end diastolic volume: Length–tension relationship

Frank-Starling mechanism of the heart. Within physiological limits, the heart pumps all the blood that comes to it without allowing excessive damming of blood in the veins.

Cardiac output regulation is the sum of all local blood flow regulations and body metabolism regulates most local blood flows. Thus CO is determined by the sum of various factors throughout the body that control the local blood flow.

Stretching of the heart results in stretching of the SA node. This has direct effect on rhythmicity of the node and heart rate increases by 10–15 per cent. Stretching of right atrium elicits Bainbridge reflex with increased heart rate.

HOMOMETRIC REGULATION (Fig. 8.2)

Sympathetic Stimulation

The cardiac accelerator action of sympathetic stimulation is known as *positive chronotropic action.*

When the strength of contraction of the heart increases without increase in fibre length, then more of the blood that normally remains in the ventricles is expelled, ejection fraction increases and end-systolic ventricular blood volume decreases. This is known as *positive inotropic action of sympathetic stimulation.*

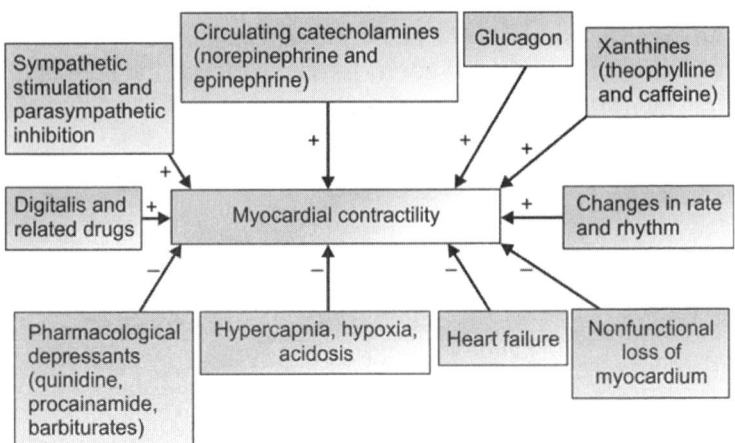

Fig. 8.2: Factors affecting myocardial contractility

Factors that increase the force of contraction are said to have positive inotropic effect. Factors that decrease the force of contraction of the heart are said to have negative inotropic effect. Force of contraction is dependent on preloading and after-loading conditions. During isometric contraction, the length of the muscle fibre remains the same and tension increases till the load is lifted.

Afterload

In isotonic contraction, the tension remains same. Shortening occurs as load is lifted and external work is performed.

An experiment can be performed in which the muscle strip is stretched by a load (preload) that rests on a platform. The elastic component in series with the contractile element is stretched and the tension increases till it is sufficient to lift the load. The tension at which the load is lifted is the *afterload*. The muscle then contracts isotonically without developing further tension. Experimentally the muscle strip can be fixed at increasing lengths and it is observed that the tension developed and the load lifted gradually increase till optimal length.

Under *in vivo* conditions, preload is the degree to which myocardium is stretched, i. e. degree of filling before it contracts.

Afterload is the resistance or the aortic pressure against which blood is expelled by the left ventricle into the aorta.

POSITIVE AND NEGATIVE INOTROPIC AGENTS

Circulating catecholamines act on adrenergic receptors and Gs (G-protein), with activation of adenylyl cyclase resulting in increased intracellular cyclic-AMP, protein kinase A phosphorylation and increased Ca^{2+} availability.

Xanthines such as caffeine and theophylline, inhibit the breakdown of cyclic-AMP and are positively inotropic.

Glucagon is positively inotropic. It increases the formation of cyclic-AMP.

Digitalis and related drugs have inhibitory effect on the Na^+-K^+ ATPase in the myocardium. This inhibition causes an

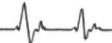

increase in intracellular Na^+ and increased availability of Ca^{2+} in the cell.

Ventricular extrasystoles affect myocardial contractility. Due to increased availability of intracellular Ca^{2+}, there is post-extrasystolic potentiation.

FACTORS THAT AFFECT AORTIC PRESSURE (AFTERLOAD), FORCE VELOCITY RELATIONSHIP

$$\text{Cardiac output} = \frac{\text{Arterial pressure}}{\text{Total peripheral resistance}}$$

Cardiac output varies inversely with total peripheral resistance, when the arterial pressure is constant.

When the aortic pressure, i.e. afterload is increased, the force or the tension developed increases during the isometric contraction to a maximum value. The number of cycling cross-bridges increases. The sliding of the filaments past each other is slow, or in other words, velocity of shortening decreases. After attaining a maximum value, no further increase in tension can occur with further increase in afterload, i. e. aortic pressure and the ejection through the aortic valve ceases.

Conversely, at zero load, the velocity of shortening is maximum, as the filaments slide past each other quickly. This is known as *force velocity relationship*.

Heart Lung Preparation

The effect of changes in peripheral resistance can be demonstrated in the heart lung preparation. The heart and lungs of an anaesthetised dog are cannulated in such a way that blood from the aorta flows through a system of tubings and a reservoir to the right atrium, through the animal's heart and lungs back to the aorta. As the heart is functionally denervated, the heart rate varies very little. By decreasing the caliber of outflow tubing, the peripheral resistance can be varied. Similarly, by adjusting the position of the reservoir, the effect of changes in venous return can be demonstrated.

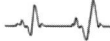

Heart Rate

Various factors increase or decrease heart rate (Figs 8.3A and B) and thus influence the cardiac output.

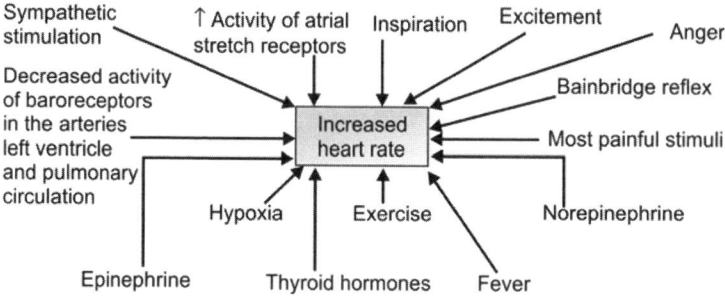

Fig. 8.3A: Factors affecting heart rate: Positive chronotropic agents

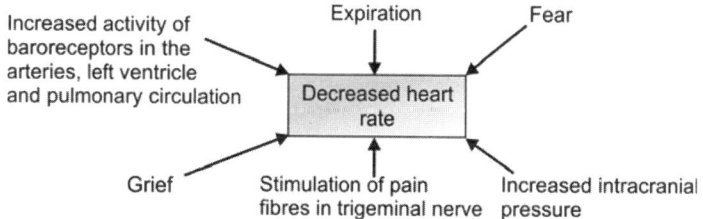

Fig. 8.3B: Negative chronotropic agents

STARLING'S CURVES OR VENTRICULAR FUNCTION CURVES AND CARDIAC OUTPUT CURVES

Cardiac function can be assessed and expressed in terms of curves relating end-diastolic volume or end-diastolic pressure or atrial pressure (which forms the central venous pressure) to stroke volume or stroke work output or cardiac output.

One can generate a family of Starling's curves at a given EDV by changing the contractility or afterload. Increasing the contractility and a decrease in afterload will shift the curve upward, because at a given EDV or atrial pressure the cells can shorten down further on the preload. The functional ability of left or right ventricle can be expressed by plotting left or right ventricular stroke work output or ventricular volume output on Y-axis against left or right atrial pressure respectively on X-axis. These two types of ventricular function curves express the function of each ventricle separately.

By fixing the variables, i.e. contractility, afterload and heart rate, the cardiac output can be plotted on the Y-axis and the preload, i.e. right atrial pressure on the X-axis and one can relate these two variables. These curves are known as *cardiac function curves or cardiac output curves* and are plotted for assessing the function of entire heart. The plateau level of normal cardiac output curve is about 12.5 L/min, 2.5 times the normal cardiac output. This is the limitation for the normal heart, without any excess nervous stimulation.

HYPEREFFECTIVE HEART (Fig. 8.4)

Factors which make the Heart Function as a Better Pump than Normal

1. *Sympathetic stimulation and parasympathetic inhibition:*
   a. Increase the heart rate to 180–200 beats/min
   b. Increase the strength of heart contraction (contractility) to twice its normal strength. The plateau level is thus doubled to 25 L/min.
2. *Heart hypertrophy:* The heart that is subjected to increased workload causes heart muscle to increase in mass and contractile strength. With nervous stimulation and heart hypertrophy, heart can be made to pump 30–40 L/min.

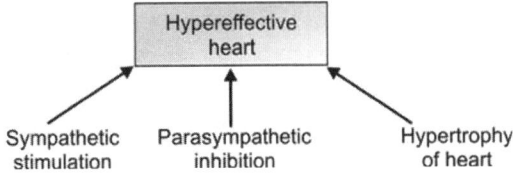

Fig. 8.4: Hypereffective heart

Pathological conditions that cause high cardiac output are always caused by reduced peripheral resistance, e.g. beriberi, anaemia, hyperthyroidism and arteriovenous fistula.

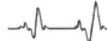

FACTORS THAT CAUSE HYPOEFFECTIVE HEART (Fig. 8.5)

Pathological Conditions that cause Low Cardiac Output

1. *Decreased pumping effectiveness of heart:*
   - i. Myocardial infarction
   - ii. Myocarditis
   - iii. Cardiac tamponade
   - iv. Severe valvular heart disease

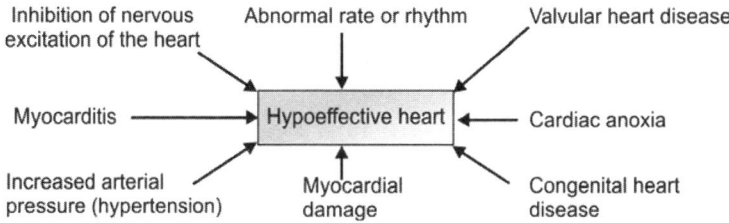

Fig. 8.5: Hypoeffective heart

2. *Decreased venous return:*
   - i. Decreased blood volume
   - ii. Acute venous dilatation
   - iii. Obstruction of large veins

PRINCIPAL FACTORS AFFECTING VENOUS RETURN

1. *Right atrial pressure:* This is the pressure, which impedes blood flow into the right atrium by exerting backward force on the veins.
2. *Mean systemic filling pressure:* This is defined as the pressure measured everywhere in the systemic circulation, when all the blood flow is stopped. This is the pressure, which forces blood towards heart (7 mmHg).
3. *Resistance to blood flow:* This is the resistance encountered to blood flow between peripheral blood vessels and the right atrium.

Venous Return Curves

These are also known as vascular curves. These curves relate right atrial pressure to the venous return.

Right Atrial Pressure (RAP)

The rising RAP exerts backward force on the venous return and causes damming of blood in the distensible systemic circulation. If all the circulatory reflexes are prevented from acting, venous return decreases to zero at a right atrial pressure of 7 mmHg. As venous return decreases to zero, the pumping by the failing heart also decreases and the arterial pressure comes to equilibrium with the venous pressure. The flow in systemic circulation stops at this pressure known as *mean systemic filling pressure.*

Plateau in the Venous Return Curve

As the right atrial pressure falls below zero, the venous return increases slightly and by the time it reaches –2 mmHg, the venous return has already reached plateau. There is no increase in the venous return even if the right atrial pressure falls further (–20 to –50 mmHg), as the negative pressure sucks the walls of the veins, where they enter the chest. Also, the atmospheric pressure causes the flaccid veins outside the chest to collapse.

Mean Systemic Filling Pressure (Psf)

When the large vessels at the base of the heart are clamped, the blood flow stops and the pressure measured everywhere in systemic circulation becomes same. This is known as *mean systemic filling pressure.* This equilibrated pressure (7 mmHg), measured everywhere in systemic circulation is independent from that of pulmonary circulation. With increase in the mean systemic filling pressure, the venous return curve shifts upward and to the right. If the mean systemic filling pressure decreases, the curve shifts downward and to the left.

Mean Circulatory Filling Pressure

When the pumping by the heart is stopped by electric shock, causing ventricular fibrillation, the flow of blood stops everywhere in the circulation a few seconds later. The pressures equilibrate everywhere in the circulation and this pressure is called *mean circulatory filling pressure.* The value is same as mean systemic filling pressure for all practical purposes, though mean circulatory filling pressure takes into account both pulmonary and systemic circulation.

At a volume of 5000 ml, the mean circulatory filling pressure is 7 mmHg. The mean circulatory filling pressure decreases to zero at a blood volume of 4000 ml. This is the unstressed volume of circulation. With strong stimulation of sympathetic system, all systemic blood vessels, larger pulmonary vessels and chambers of heart constrict, reducing the capacity of the system. Hence at each blood volume, the mean circulatory filling pressure increases, as the vascular capacity is decreased.

Thus strong sympathetic stimulation increases the mean systemic circulatory filling pressure to 17 mmHg at normal blood volume and complete sympathetic inhibition decreases this to 4 mmHg. The difference between the mean systemic filling pressure and right atrial pressure is known as the pressure gradient for venous return. The pressure gradient is zero when venous return becomes zero (RAP equals Psf).

Resistance to Venous Return

Most of the resistance to venous return occurs in the veins (2/3rd) and some in the arterioles and small arteries (1/3rd). When the resistance in the veins increases, blood begins to be dammed up in all parts of systemic circulation. As the veins are highly distensible, the damming up of blood in the veins causes negligible increase in the venous pressure. Thus the resistance is not overcome and venous return decreases. On the other hand, the arteries being less distensible and having 1/30th the capacitance of veins, any increase in resistance to flow results in significant increase in pressure and subsequently flow.

Venous return is given by the formula:

$$VR = \frac{Psf - RAP}{RVR}$$

$$= \frac{7 - 0 \text{ mmHg}}{1.4 \text{ mmHg} / L}$$

$$= 5 \text{ L} / \min$$

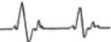

METHODS OF MEASURING CARDIAC OUTPUT

In Animals

Electromagnetic flowmeter can be placed on ascending aorta and the blood flow can be measured. One can cannulate aorta, pulmonary artery or great veins and measure cardiac output using any type of flowmeter.

In Humans

1. Doppler combined with echocardiography
2. Direct Fick's method
3. Indicator dilution method including thermodilution technique
4. Nuclear magnetic resonance (NMR).

Fick's Method

Fick's principle states that the amount of a substance taken up by an organ or by the whole body, per unit time, is equal to the arterial level of the substance minus the venous level (AV difference), times the blood flow.

Cardiac output can be measured by measuring the amount of O_2 consumed by the body in a given period of time and dividing this value by the arteriovenous difference across the lungs. As systemic arterial blood has the same O_2 content all over the body, arterial sample can be obtained from any convenient artery. A mixed venous blood sample is obtained from pulmonary artery by means of a cardiac catheter. The catheter is inserted through forearm vein, its tip being guided into the heart with the aid of a fluoroscope.

Cardiac catheterisation was first attempted in 1929 by Dr Werner Forssman, a resident doctor in a hospital from a place near Berlin. He was the first one to attempt cardiac catheterisation, himself being the subject. He practised cardiac catheterisation on himself nine times but the medical world was not convinced of the safety of the procedure. It was only 27 years later that his merit was recognized and was awarded Nobel Prize for Physiology and Medicine jointly with Dr Andre F Cournand and Dr Dickinson W Richards in 1956.

$$\text{Output of left ventricle} = \frac{O_2 \text{ Consumption (ml/min)}}{(AO_2) - (VO_2)}$$

Indicator Dilution Technique

A known amount of substance (a dye or more commonly a radioactive isotope) is injected into an arm vein and the concentration of the substance in serial samples of arterial blood is determined every 2 seconds. The log of the indicator concentration in the serial arterial samples is plotted against time. The concentration initially rises, then falls and rises again as the indicator recirculates. The single circulation time (Y seconds) is the time for the first passage of the indicator through the circulation, which is obtained by extrapolating initial decline in the concentration to the abscissa. The output during the single circulation time is given by:

$$\text{Flow in 'Y' seconds} = \frac{\text{Amount of indicator injected (E)}}{\text{Average concentration of the indicator (C)}}$$

The average concentration of the indicator can be calculated from the serial concentrations of the indicator obtained every two seconds.

Cardiac output is calculated as:

$$\text{Flow per minute} = \frac{E}{(C)} \times \frac{60}{Y} L$$

The indicator must be:
1. A substance that stays in the bloodstream during the test.
2. Has no harmful or haemodynamic effects.
3. Its concentration in the blood should be easy to measure.

Thermodilution Technique

The indicator used is cold saline. The cold saline is injected into right atrium through one side of a double lumen catheter and the temperature change in the blood in the pulmonary artery is recorded using a thermistor, located in the other longer side of the catheter. The temperature change is inversely proportional to the amount of blood flowing through the pulmonary artery, i.e. to the extent that the cold saline is diluted by blood.

Advantages

1. Saline is not harmful.
2. Recirculation is not a problem as cold is dissipated in tissues.
3. It is easy to make repeated measurements.

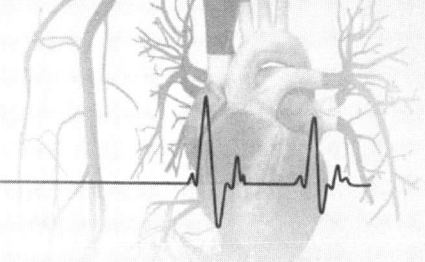

9

Arterial Pressure

DEFINITIONS

The pressure in the aorta and in large arteries rises to a peak value (systolic pressure, 110–120 mmHg) and falls to a minimum value (diastolic pressure, 70–80 mmHg) during each heart cycle.

PULSE PRESSURE

The difference between systolic and diastolic pressure is 40–50 mmHg and is known as pulse pressure.

Pulse Pressure Depends Upon

1. The stroke volume output of the heart
2. The compliance, i. e. total distensibility of the arterial tree

MEAN ARTERIAL PRESSURE

The average pressure throughout the cardiac cycle is known as *mean arterial pressure*. As systole is shorter than diastole, mean pressure is slightly less than the value halfway between systolic and diastolic pressure.

Mean arterial pressure is diastolic pressure plus one-third of the pulse pressure as an approximation. The arterial pressure falls slightly in large and medium-sized arteries. The arterial pressure falls rapidly in small arteries and arterioles, which are the main sites of peripheral resistance. At the ends of arterioles, the mean pressure is 30–38 mmHg. Pulse pressure also declines to about 5 mmHg at the ends of arterioles.

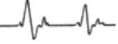

NORMAL ARTERIAL PRESSURE

The arterial pressure in the brachial artery in young adults, in the sitting or lying position at rest, is approximately 120/80 mmHg (systolic/diastolic). It is lower at night and lower in women. As it is a product of cardiac output (CO) and total peripheral resistance (TPR), conditions that affect CO or TPR affect arterial pressure. Generally, conditions that increase CO increase systolic pressure and conditions that increase TPR increase diastolic pressure. With age, both increase.

EFFECT OF GRAVITY

The pressures described are those at heart level. The pressure in any vessel above the heart level decreases and below the heart level increases due to effect of gravity. The product of density of blood, acceleration due to gravity (980 cm/s/s), vertical distance above or below the heart is 0.77 mmHg/cm of column of blood. When the mean arterial pressure is 100 mmHg at heart level, the mean pressure in a large artery, 40 cm above, in the head will be $100 - (0.77 \times 40) = 69$ mmHg.

METHODS OF MEASURING ARTERIAL PRESSURE

In an experimental animal, a cannula can be inserted into an artery and the artery can be tied off beyond this point. The *end pressure* can be measured by connecting this cannula to a mercury manometer, or a suitably calibrated strain gauge and an oscillograph, which writes on a moving strip of paper. When a "T" tube is inserted into the vessel, the pressure measured in the side arm of the tube is *side pressure*. This side pressure is lower than the end pressure, by the kinetic energy of flow, where the pressure drop due to resistance is negligible.

As per Bernoulli's principle, in a tube or a blood vessel, the total energy, i.e. the sum of kinetic energy of flow and the pressure energy is constant. In any segment of arterial system, the pressure drop is both due to resistance and to conversion of potential into kinetic energy. The pressure drop due to energy lost in overcoming resistance is irreversible as it is dissipated as heat. When a vessel narrows, more of the potential energy is converted to kinetic energy of flow, the velocity of flow increases and the lateral pressure on the walls decreases. Thus the narrowing tends to maintain itself. However, pressure drop that results due to conversion of potential to kinetic energy (as a vessel narrows) is reversed, when the vessel widens out again.

Palpation Method

An inflatable arm cuff (Riva-Rocci cuff) is tied around the arm and the pressure in the sphygmomanometer is increased to a value till radial pulse disappears. The pressure is decreased gradually and the pressure at which radial pulse first becomes palpable is noted. This is *systolic pressure*. Pressures obtained by this method are usually 2–5 mmHg lower than those obtained by auscultatory method.

Auscultatory gap: The sounds of Korotkoff sometimes disappear at pressures above diastolic pressure. They then reappear at lower pressures. This is known as *auscultatory gap*. Thus, the value of diastolic pressure recorded is higher than the actual diastolic pressure. This can be avoided, if the cuff is inflated till the radial pulse disappears.

Auscultatory Method

The arterial pressure in humans is measured by auscultatory method. An inflatable cuff (Riva-Rocci cuff), attached to sphygmomanometer, is wrapped around the arm at the heart level. The stethoscope is placed over the brachial artery. The cuff is inflated well above the expected systolic pressure, recorded through palpation method. At this point, as the artery is occluded, no sound is heard. The cuff pressure is now lowered slowly and at a point when the systolic pressure in the artery just exceeds the cuff pressure, blood passes through at the peak of the systole with each heartbeat and a tapping sound is heard. As the pressure is gradually lowered, the sounds become louder, then dull, muffled and finally they disappear. The value at which the sounds disappear is taken as diastolic pressure. These are the sounds of *Korotkoff* and are produced by turbulent flow in the brachial artery.

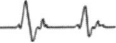

Explanation

Streamline flow is silent. When the artery is constricted, the velocity of flow exceeds critical velocity and turbulence occurs. Tapping sound is produced by intermittent turbulence at the peak of systole. When the cuff pressure is above diastolic pressure in the artery, flow is interrupted during part of diastole. The intermittent sounds have *staccato* quality. The vessel is still constricted when the cuff pressure is near the arterial diastolic pressure, but the turbulent flow is continuous and has the muffled quality. Ultimately the sounds disappear and this is taken as diastolic pressure.

Precautions

1. Wider cuff should be used in obese persons
2. Cuff should be tied at heart level
3. Cuff, if left inflated, causes reflex vasoconstriction
4. Blood pressure should be compared in both arms

Pressure Pulses and their Transmission

The blood ejected into the aorta during systole distends the proximal portion of the aorta initially. The blood does not move to periphery due to inertia. The rising pressure in the aorta overcomes the inertia and the wave of distention spreads along the aorta gradually. This is known as *transmission of pressure pulse* in the arteries.

Velocity of pressure pulse transmission is inversely proportional to the compliance of the vessels. In aorta, it is 3–5 m/s. In large arterial branches, it is 7–10 m/s. In small arteries, it is 15–35 m/s. The pressure pulse is a moving wave of pressure that involves a little forward movement of blood volume. Hence, in aorta, the velocity of transmission of pressure pulse is greater than the velocity of blood flow.

By the time blood reaches the capillaries, the intensity of pulsations diminishes gradually and the pressure pulsations are reduced to no pulsations. The blood flow becomes continuous in the tissues. This occurs due to:

1. The resistance to blood movement in the vessels
2. The compliance of the vessels

This is called *damping of the pressure pulses.*

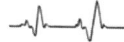

VASCULAR DISTENSIBILITY

Vascular distensibility is defined as fractional increase in volume, for each millimetre of mercury rise in pressure.

$$\frac{\text{Vascular}}{\text{distensibility}} = \frac{\text{Increase in volume}}{\text{Increase in pressure} \times \text{Original volume}}$$

The pressure pulsations due to pulsatile output of the heart are averaged out by the distensible nature of arteries and veins. This provides an almost completely smooth, continuous flow of blood through the small blood vessels of the tissues. The veins are the most distensible vessels.

Pulmonary arteries operate at pressures one-sixth those in systemic circulation and have six times the distensibility of systemic arteries.

VASCULAR COMPLIANCE OR CAPACITANCE

The total quantity of blood that can be stored in a given portion of circulation, for each millimetre of mercury rise in pressure is known as *vascular compliance or capacitance.*

$$\text{Vascular compliance} = \frac{\text{Increase in volume}}{\text{Increase in pressure}}$$

Compliance is equal to distensibility times volume. A vessel having slight volume has less compliance, though it is highly distensible than a vessel, which has large volume but is less distensible. The compliance of a vein is 24 times that of its corresponding artery.

NERVOUS REGULATION OF CIRCULATION

Vasomotor Centre (VMC) and Vasoconstrictor System

The vasomotor centre is located bilaterally in the reticular substance of the medulla and lower third of pons. The VMC transmits sympathetic impulses through the spinal cord and peripheral sympathetic nerves to almost all blood vessels of the body. Parasympathetic impulses are transmitted from the centre through vagus nerve to the heart.

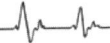
Autonomic Nervous System

Sympathetic
Thoracolumbar outflow from spinal cord to sympathetic chain gives rise to:
1. Specific sympathetic nerves that innervate the vasculature of internal viscera and the heart
2. Spinal nerves that innervate the vasculature of peripheral areas.

All the vessels are innervated except the capillaries, precapillary sphincters and most of the meta-arterioles.

When the small arteries and arterioles constrict, they increase the resistance to blood flow and thereby decrease the rate of blood flow through the tissues.

Sympathetic stimulation of veins decreases the volume of these vessels and alters the volume of the peripheral circulation. Thus blood translocates into the heart.

VASOMOTOR CENTRE (Fig. 9.1)

The vasomotor centre is a diffuse area in the reticular formation. It consists of:
1. **Vasoconstrictor area (C1):** It is bilaterally located in the anterolateral portions of upper medulla. Their fibres are distributed throughout the cord (bulbospinal), in the inter-mediolateral gray column of the spinal cord. They leave the spinal cord through all thoracic and the first one or two lumbar spinal nerves, to the paravertebral sympathetic chain and relay in the sympathetic ganglia. Postganglionic fibres pass on to the blood vessels in the viscera. Glutamate is released as neurotransmitter.
2. **Vasodilator area (A1):** Located bilaterally in the anterolateral portions of the lower half of medulla, the fibres project upwards and inhibit C1 causing vasodilation. GABA is the neurotransmitter.
3. **Sensory area (A2):** Located bilaterally in the nucleus of the tractus solitarius and in the posterolateral portions of the medulla and lower pons, sensory signals are received from vagus and glossopharyngeal nerves and output signals

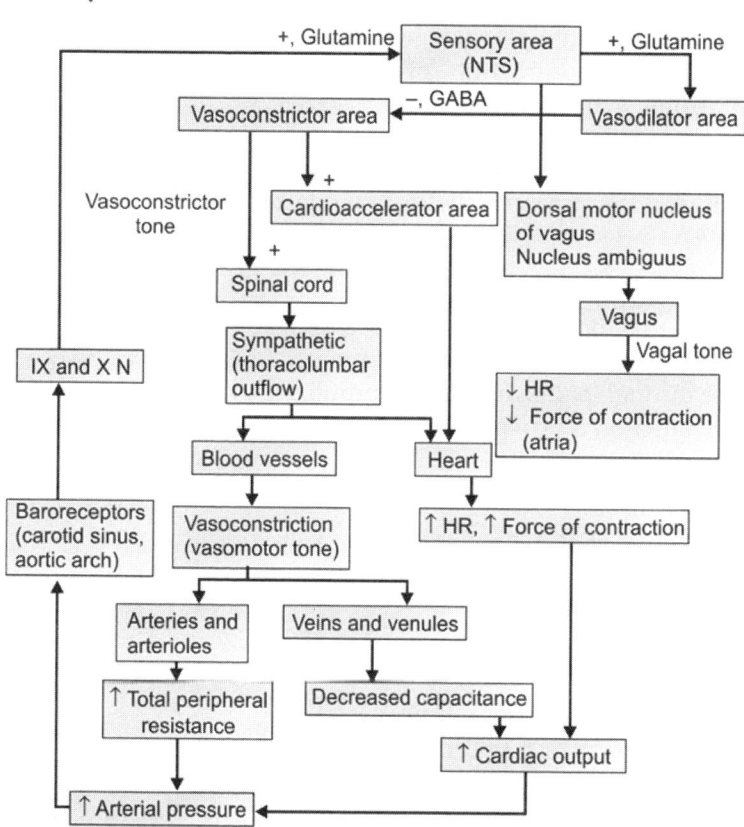

Fig. 9.1: Vasomotor centre

control activities of vasoconstrictor and vasodilator areas of the vasomotor centre. It brings about control of many reflexes, e.g. baroreceptor reflex for controlling arterial pressure.

Cardioaccelerator Area

The lateral portions of VMC transmit excitatory impulses through sympathetic nerve fibres to the heart, to increase heart rate and contractility. This is *cardioaccelerator area*. Vasoconstriction and cardiac acceleration go hand in hand.

The sympathetic nerve fibres to the heart increase heart rate and force of contraction (positive chronotropic and positive inotropic action). The sympathetic nerves carry tremendous numbers of vasoconstrictor fibres and only a few vasodilator fibres. Their distribution is greater in kidneys, gut, spleen and skin and less potent in skeletal muscle and brain.

Cardioinhibitory Area

The medial portion of VMC, lying in close apposition to dorsal motor nucleus of vagus, when stimulated causes decrease in heart rate through parasympathetic impulses carried through vagus. Vasodilation is brought about by inhibition of vasoconstriction or vasoconstrictor tone.

Parasympathetic Control of Heart Function

Vagal stimulation (negative chronotropic action) decreases mainly heart rate.

SYMPATHETIC VASOCONSTRICTOR TONE AND VASOMOTOR TONE

The vasoconstrictor area of the VMC transmits signals continuously to the sympathetic vasoconstrictor fibres over the entire body, causing continuous slow firing of the fibres at a rate of about ½–2 impulses per second. This is known as the *sympathetic vasoconstrictor tone*. These impulses maintain the blood vessels in a partial state of contraction called *vasomotor tone*. The neurotransmitter secreted by sympathetic vasoconstrictor fibres is norepinephrine. It acts on the alpha receptors of the vascular smooth muscle to cause *vasoconstriction*.

Sympathetic impulses are transmitted simultaneously to the adrenal medullae, as they are transmitted to all blood vessels. The medullae secrete both epinephrine and norepinephrine, which circulate in the blood and cause direct vasoconstriction. Sometimes due to its potent beta receptor action, epinephrine causes vasodilation.

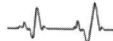

SYMPATHETIC VASODILATOR SYSTEM (Fig. 9.2) AND ITS IMPORTANCE

Though the sympathetic nerves carry predominantly vasoconstrictor fibres, the sympathetic nerves to skeletal muscles carry both vasodilator and constrictor fibres. The neurotransmitter released at the nerve endings of vasodilator fibres in cats is acetylcholine (hence the name is given as sympathetic cholinergic vasodilator system). However, in primates, epinephrine may be causing the vasodilation through beta receptor action. Anterior hypothalamus controls this area.

The importance of this system in human beings is not well understood. However, it plays possible role in the following:

1. At the onset of exercise, even before the muscles actually require increased quantity of nutrients, the sympathetic vasodilator system might cause anticipatory increase in blood flow.

2. *Emotional fainting-vasovagal syncope:* Some people experience severe emotional disturbance that causes fainting due to intense vasodilation. This is known as *vasovagal syncope or emotional fainting.*

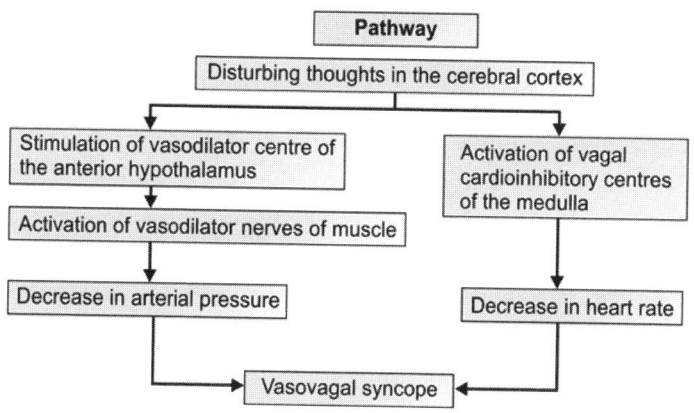

Fig. 9.2: Sympathetic vasodilator system

REGULATION OF ACTIVITY OF VASOMOTOR CENTRE (Fig. 9.3)

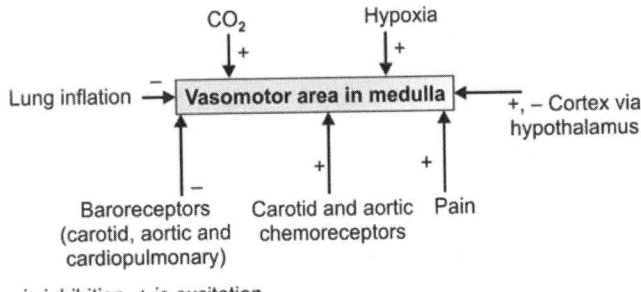

Fig. 9.3: Regulation of vasomotor centre

INFLUENCE OF HIGHER CENTRES ON VASOMOTOR CENTRE

Large number of areas in the reticular substance of pons, mesencephalon and diencephalon can either excite or inhibit vasomotor centre. Descending fibres/tracts from cerebral cortex, particularly the limbic cortex, relay in hypothalamus and then pass onto vasomotor centre. Emotions such as anger, sexual excitement, etc. cause rise in blood pressure and tachycardia. Posterolateral portions of the hypothalamus cause mainly excitation, whereas anterior portions can cause inhibition or mild excitation.

ARTERIAL PRESSURE REGULATION

1. *Rapidly acting pressure control mechanisms* (act rapidly within seconds/minutes):
   a. Baroreceptor
   b. CNS ischaemic response
   c. Chemoreceptor mechanism
2. *Intermediate control mechanisms* (respond from 30 minutes to several hours):
   a. The renin-angiotensin vasoconstrictor system
   b. Stress relaxation of vessels
   c. Capillary fluid shift

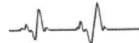

3. *Long-term control mechanisms* (provide regulation over days, months and years):
   a. Renal body fluid pressure control mechanisms
   b. Aldosterone secretion

RAPID CONTROL OF ARTERIAL PRESSURE

Rapid control of arterial pressure is brought about by stimulation of sympathetic nervous system and reciprocal inhibition of parasympathetic, vagal inhibitory signals to the heart. The vasoconstrictor and the cardioaccelerator functions of the sympathetic nervous system are stimulated as a unit.

As a result:

1. All the arterioles are constricted→↑total peripheral resistance, ↑arterial pressure
2. The veins and other larger vessels of circulation are strongly constricted→translocation of blood towards heart→– ↑volume of blood returning to the heart→↑pumping and↑arterial pressure
3. Increase in heart rate (3 times normal), increase in contractility→↑output (25 L/min) →↑in arterial pressure

Arterial pressure increases within seconds (5–10) to twice the normal. Sudden inhibition of nervous stimulation can cause pressure to fall to half the normal value within 10–40 seconds.

BARORECEPTORS

There are special subconscious nervous control mechanisms maintaining the arterial pressure. These are the negative feedback reflex mechanisms.

Baroreceptors are stretch receptors. They are knobby, coiled, extensively branched and intertwined spray type endings of myelinated nerve fibres, located in the walls of large systemic arteries. A few baroreceptors are present in the wall of almost every large artery of the thoracic and neck region.

→ leading to; ↑ increase

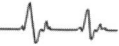

They are extremely abundant in:

1. The wall of carotid sinus, which is a dilated portion of each internal carotid artery, slightly above the carotid bifurcation
2. The wall of aortic arch.

Pathway for the Afferent Impulses

- Carotid sinus → Hering's nerve → glossopharyngeal nerve → tractus solitarius in the medulla of the brainstem
- Aortic arch → vagus → tractus solitarius

RESPONSES OF BARORECEPTORS TO PRESSURE CHANGES

1. The baroreceptors are not stimulated much in the pressure range of 0–60 mmHg. They respond progressively more rapidly above 60 mmHg and reach maximum at 180 mmHg. Aortic receptors operate at 30 mmHg higher pressure levels.
2. The rate of baroreceptor firing increases during systole and decreases during diastole.
3. Baroreceptors respond much more rapidly to changing pressures than to stationary pressures.
4. They operate with maximum sensitivity in the normal operating range of arterial pressure, i. e. around 100 mmHg.
5. If the arterial pressure changes last more than a few days, baroreceptors adapt quickly.
6. They are responsible for preventing rapid changes in arterial pressure, coming into play within seconds. If the change in arterial pressure persists for 1–2 days, the baroreceptors reset at the new pressure and the number of impulses passing through them (impulse rate firing) decreases to normal, despite the elevated pressure.
7. *Buffer function:* Baroreceptors maintain the arterial pressure in the range of 85–115 mmHg, throughout the day. When the carotid and aortic baroreceptors are denervated, there are wide fluctuations in arterial pressure with day-to-day activities. Hence, baroreceptors are known as *pressure buffer system* and the nerves from them are known as *buffer nerves.*

→ leading to

8. Baroreceptors maintain the arterial pressure constant with changes in body posture. There is marked fall in the arterial pressure in the head and upper part of the body on standing. This falling pressure inactivates baroreceptors and their inhibitory effect on vasomotor centre is lost. The sympathetic nervous system is stimulated and the decrease in pressure is minimized.

BARORECEPTOR REFLEX

Increase in arterial pressure→ stretching of the wall of the carotid sinus and aortic arch and hence the baroreceptors→ baroreceptor signals enter the nucleus tractus solitarius through IXth and Xth cranial nerves→ inhibition of vasoconstrictor centre and stimulation of vagal centre resulting in:

1. Vasodilation of veins, arterioles, throughout the peripheral circulatory system
2. Decrease in heart rate and strength of contraction→ ↓cardiac output and peripheral resistance.

On the other hand, if both common carotids are clamped or ligated→ ↓carotid sinus pressure→ baroreceptors inactive→ inhibitory effect on vasomotor centre is lost→↑in arterial pressure occurs, which remains so during the period the carotids are occluded.

Slight over compensation occurs when the carotids are released.

Carotid and Aortic Chemoreceptors

Chemoreceptors operate in 40–80 mmHg arterial pressure range. Whenever the arterial pressure falls, the blood flow to chemoreceptors and the availability of oxygen decrease. The CO_2 and hydrogen ions build up in excess and the chemoreceptors are stimulated. The *vasomotor centre* is stimulated leading to increase in the arterial pressure. Chemoreceptor reflex is a powerful arterial pressure controller, when the arterial pressure falls below 80 mmHg.

→ leads to; ↓ decrease; ↑ increase

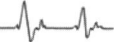
CENTRAL NERVOUS SYSTEM ISCHAEMIC RESPONSE

Decreased blood flow to vasomotor centre → neurons become strongly excited due to:
1. Cerebral ischaemia
2. Failure of the slowly flowing blood to carry away CO_2 and other metabolites from vasomotor centre → stimulation of sympathetic vasoconstrictor system→intense vasoconstriction all over the body due to intense cerebral ischaemia.

The arterial pressure is elevated to 250 mmHg or so for 10 minutes. This is the most powerful of all the stimulatory mechanisms of sympathetic vasoconstrictor system and is known as *central nervous system ischaemic response.*

When arterial pressure decreases to <60 mmHg, it starts operating. The response is highest at 15–20 mmHg. It is an emergency arterial pressure control system and is sometimes called *last ditch stand* pressure control mechanism.

If cerebral ischaemia is so severe that increase in arterial pressure cannot relieve it, the neuronal cells become inactive within 3–10 minutes and die in 20–60 minutes time. When the arterial pressure decreases to 40–50 mmHg → vasomotor centre loses all its activity.

CUSHING REACTION

Increase in CSF pressure compresses the arteries→cuts off blood supply to the brain→CNS ischaemic response→↑arterial pressure→blood flows again→ischaemia relieved. Whenever CSF pressure rises, Cushing reaction helps to protect the vital centres of the brain.

VARIOUS OTHER REFLEXES

Atrial Receptors and Atrial Reflexes

Located in the atrial walls, there are 2 types of stretch receptors.

Type A receptors: Discharge primarily in atrial systole.

Type B receptors: These are volume receptors or low pressure receptors. They cannot detect changes in the systemic arterial

---

→ leads to; ↓ decrease; ↑ increase

pressure. However, they detect simultaneous increase in pressure in the low pressure areas of circulation, caused by an increase in volume. The volume reflexes are parallel to the baroreceptor reflexes.

Atrial Reflexes to Kidneys

↓*ECF volume* → ↓*central venous pressure*→ ↓*firing of atrial stretch receptors (B type):*

1. Increased secretion of vasopressin from hypothalamus
2. Increased sympathetic activity→↑secretion of renin→ ↑secretion of aldosterone→ net result is retention of fluid and sodium.

On the other hand, when the volume load to the atria increases:

Stretch of the atria → *increased firing of atrial type B stretch receptors:*

1. Dilation of afferent arterioles in the kidneys→decreased afferent arteriolar resistance→↑glomerular capillary pressure→↑filtration of fluid into kidney tubules.
2. Signals are transmitted simultaneously to hypothalamus→ ↓ ADH→ ↓reabsorption of water from tubules.
3. Atrial natriuretic peptide secreted from atrial muscle cells→ acts on kidney resulting in loss of Na^+ → rapid loss of fluid.

Thus blood volume is controlled and arterial pressure is brought back to normal.

Reflex control of heart rate by atria: Bainbridge reflex was discovered in 1915 by Bainbridge. With an increase in atrial pressure, the heart rate increases sometimes to as much as 75 per cent. Direct stretch of the SA node causes 15 per cent increase and the additional 40–60 per cent increase is by Bainbridge reflex. This is a true reflex. Afferent signals pass through vagus nerves to medulla and efferents through sympathetic and vagus nerves.

This reflex prevents damming of blood in the veins, atria and pulmonary circulation.

→ leads to; ↓ decrease; ↑ increase

Left Ventricular Receptors: Bezold-Jarisch Reflex or Coronary Chemoreflex

In experimental animals, injections of serotonin, veratridine, capsaicin, phenyldiguanide and some other drugs into coronary arteries supplying left ventricle cause apnoea, followed by rapid breathing, hypotension and bradycardia. The receptors are C fibre endings. The afferents are vagal. The physiological significance of this reflex is not known. It may play role in the maintenance of the vagal tone that keeps heart rate low at rest.

Pulmonary Receptors: Pulmonary Chemoreflex

In experimental animals, injections of serotonin, capsaicin, veratridine, etc. into the pulmonary artery activate C fibre endings close to the capillaries in the lungs and produce apnoea, followed by rapid breathing, hypotension and bradycardia. The wall of the pulmonary artery also has the low pressure volume receptors.

Role of Skeletal Nerves and Skeletal Muscles in Controlling Arterial Pressure

Role of abdominal muscles: Abdominal compression reflex

1. When a baroreceptor or a chemoreceptor reflex is elicited → vasomotor centre is stimulated → sympathetic vasoconstrictor system is activated → nervous impulses are transmitted to abdominal muscles →↑in basal tone of these muscles→ compresses all venous reservoirs of the abdomen→ translocation of blood towards heart → *abdominal compression reflex* is elicited.
2. When the skeletal muscles contract during exercise, the blood vessels are compressed and large quantities of blood are translocated to heart and lung. This causes increase in cardiac output and arterial pressure.
3. With heavy exercise, there is increase in blood flow and arterial pressure. The increase in blood flow is due to:

→ leads to; ↑ increase

a. *Increase in arterial pressure:* Increase in arterial pressure is due to stimulation of reticular activating system (RAS) of the brainstem along with motor areas of the cortex, resulting in stimulation of the vasoconstrictor and cardio-acceleratory areas of VMC.

b. Local vasodilation of the blood vessels of the muscle due to increase in metabolism

4. Stress reactions like alarm reaction→ arterial pressure doubles→↑ blood supply to all muscles of the body→ flight from danger.

Traube-Hering Waves

There are fluctuations in arterial pressure of 4–6 mmHg magnitude during normal respiration. There is an increase in arterial pressure during early part of expiration and a fall in pressure during remainder of respiratory cycle. With each cycle of respiration, these changes in arterial pressure are recorded in a wave-like manner, which are known as *Traube-Hering waves.*

The possible reasons for the occurrence of these waves could be:

1. Spill over of the impulses from the respiratory centre into the vasomotor centre.

2. Momentary decrease in the cardiac output and the arterial pressure with every inspiration, as the blood vessels in the chest expand with negative thoracic cavity pressure.

3. Excitation of vascular and atrial stretch receptors, with changes in pressure occurring in thoracic vessels during respiration.

Mayer Waves (Vasomotor Waves)

In experimental preparations due to oscillation of baro-receptor or chemoreceptor reflexes, there are larger fluctuations in arterial pressure as great as 10–40 mmHg, that rise and fall more slowly than the respiratory waves. Oscillation of any reflex mechanism can occur, when the response to the stimulus is not instantaneous.

→ leads to; ↑ increase

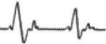

Oscillation of baroreceptor reflex

High pressure excites baroreceptors→ sympathetic nervous system inhibited→ pressure lowered a few seconds later → decreased pressure reduces the baroreceptor stimulation→ VMC active once again → pressure elevated to a high value but again the response is not instantaneous. Another cycle is initiated and oscillation continues.

Oscillation of chemoreceptor reflex

In the 40–80 mmHg pressure range, chemoreceptors control the circulation.

Haemorrhage→ hypotension → chemoreceptor drive → ↑arterial pressure. Again the response is delayed and cycle repeats.

INTERMEDIATE CONTROL MECHANISMS

1. The Renin-Angiotensin Vasoconstrictor Mechanism

When the arterial pressure falls too low, renin, a small protein enzyme, is released by the juxtaglomerular cells (JG cells) of the kidneys (Fig. 9.4).

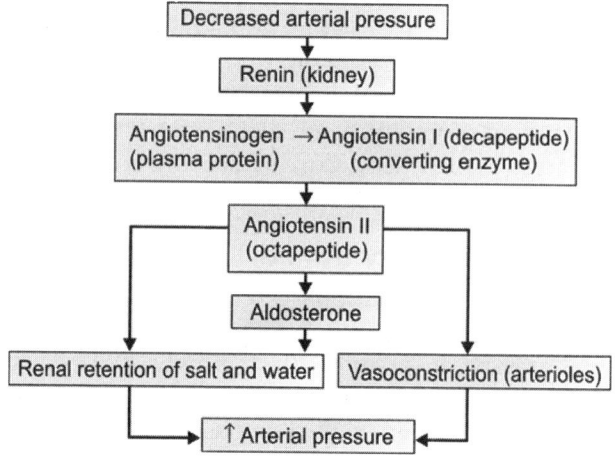

Fig. 9.4: Renin-angiotensin system

→ leads to; ↑ increase

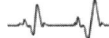

2. Stress Relaxation of Blood Vessels

Increased pressure in blood vessels→ blood vessels become stretched more and more, for minutes or hours → ↓ pressure occurs.

3. Capillary Fluid Shift

Decreased capillary pressure to low values→ fluid absorbed by osmosis from the tissue→↑ blood volume and in pressure occur.

LONG-TERM CONTROL MECHANISMS (FIG. 9.5)

When the arterial pressure changes slowly over many days, weeks or months, the kidneys come into play. Renal blood

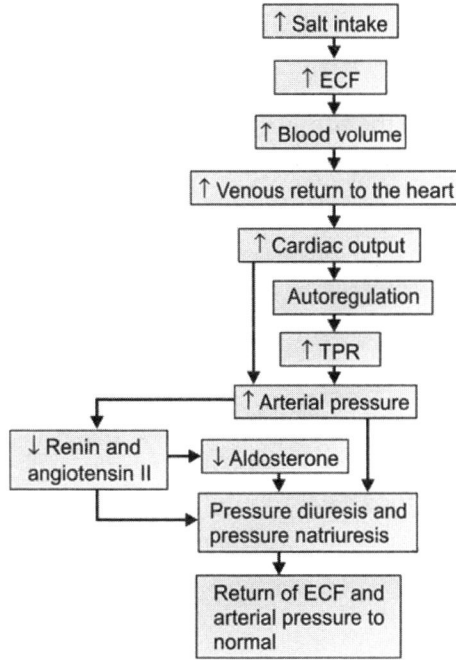

Fig. 9.5: Interaction of renin–angiotensin system with long-term control mechanisms

↑ increase; → leads to; ↓ decrease

volume–pressure control mechanism, which is same as renal body fluid–pressure control mechanism, takes a few hours to show significant response. The renal body fluid-pressure control mechanism has a feedback gain for control of arterial pressure, that equals infinity. The intake of salt and water equals salt and water output by the kidneys at the equilibrium point, at which the arterial pressure is normal. The kidneys regulate the arterial pressure precisely at this level, by increasing or decreasing the output of salt and water. Within a few hours of increase in arterial pressure by only a few millimeters of mercury, the renal output of water and salt double, which are called *pressure diuresis* and *pressure natriuresis*, respectively.

When the arterial pressure rises to about 150 mmHg, the renal output of salt and water increases to 3 times the intake, body loses fluid, blood volume decreases and arterial pressure returns to normal. On the other hand, when the arterial pressure decreases, the intake of water and salt increases more than the output, blood volume increases and arterial pressure increases, till it returns exactly to the equilibrium point. The renin-angiotensin system (angiotensin II) acts directly and through the hormone aldosterone in modifying the renal body fluid pressure system. Both angiotensin II and aldosterone increase salt and water reabsorption through kidneys (Fig. 9.5).

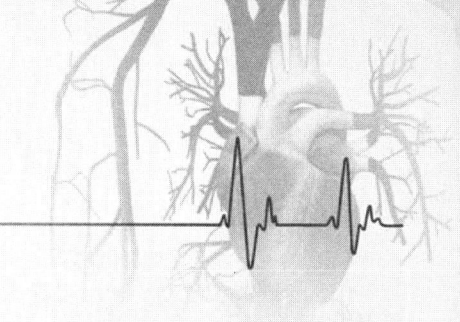

10

Heart Sounds

NORMAL HEART SOUNDS

Heart sounds are caused by closing of valves. Opening of valves does not cause any audible sound.

There are four normal heart sounds. The first and second heart sounds are audible with the help of stethoscope. The 3rd and 4th heart sounds are not audible and can be recorded as *phonocardiogram.*

First Heart Sound

At the beginning of isovolumic contraction phase, there is sudden back flow of blood against the AV valves due to contraction of ventricles, causing them to close and bulge into the atria. The elastic tautness of the chordae tendineae and the valves, keeps the valves taut, blood is prevented from moving backwards and is bounced forward causing the blood, the ventricular walls and the taut valves to vibrate. These vibrations traverse through chest wall and are heard as first heart sound by stethoscope, as "Lub". The duration is 0.14 seconds and the frequency is 25–45 Hz. It marks the beginning of isovolumic contraction phase (ventricular systole).

Second Heart Sound

It results from the closure of semilunar valves at the end of systole. At the end of ventricular systole, as the aortic/pulmonary artery pressures exceed the pressures in the left/right ventricle respectively, the blood moves backwards towards the semilunar valves for a short while. The valves bulge into the ventricles and their elastic stretch recoils the blood back and forth between these valves and the walls of arteries. These vibrations are transmitted along the chest wall and create an audible sound "Dup". It is high pitched in quality and is of 0. 11 seconds duration.

Third Heart Sound

A weak rumbling heart sound is heard at the cardiac apex sometimes with the bell of the stethoscope and is recorded in the phonocardiogram at the beginning of the middle third of diastole. It could be due to oscillation of blood back and forth between the walls of the ventricles, initiated by inrushing blood from the atria. Third heart sound is physiological in children and young adults, but usually disappears at the age of 40.

Pathologically, it occurs with high conditions output like in anaemia, fever, pregnancy and thyrotoxicosis. After 40 years of age, its occurrence is indicative of left ventricular failure, less commonly mitral regurgitation or constrictive pericarditis.

Fourth Heart Sound or Atrial Heart Sound

It is recorded in the phonocardiogram. It is very weak and has very low frequency. It occurs when the atria contract late in diastole, when blood rushes into already filled ventricles, that initiates vibrations. Fourth heart sound is sometimes physiological in the elderly. It is pathological, when it occurs with vigorous atrial contraction in hypertension, aortic stenosis, etc.

HEART MURMURS

Heart murmurs are abnormal sounds or noise heard over the heart. They are caused by turbulent flow within the heart, when the velocity of flow exceeds critical velocity. The turbulence may be caused by increased flow through a normal valve (innocent murmurs).

Pathological Conditions that Cause Murmurs

Valvular lesions due to rheumatic fever, scarring of the valves or congenital defects in the valves lead to different types of murmurs.

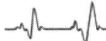

Some of the Conditions

Aortic stenosis, aortic regurgitation, mitral stenosis and mitral regurgitation.

The murmurs can be heard through stethoscope or recorded in the phonocardiogram.

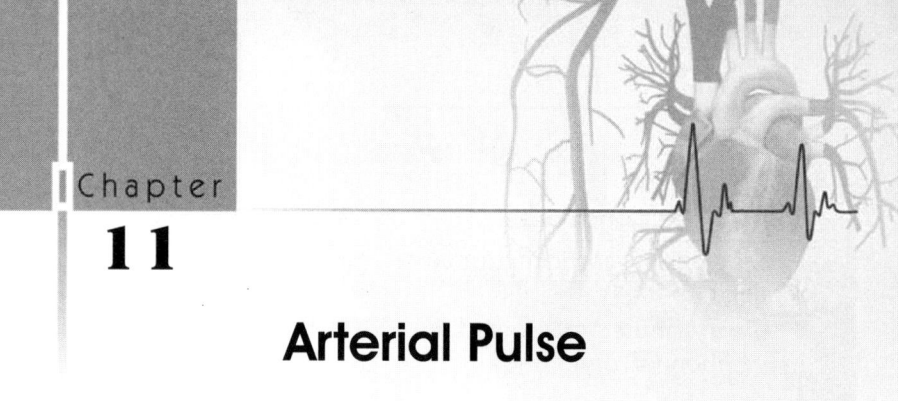

Arterial Pulse

CHARACTERISTICS

The blood ejected out into the aorta during systole moves the blood forward and sets up pressure pulsations all along the arterial tree. However, in the tissues the flow is continuous, as the compliance of the arterial tree reduces the pressure pulsations by the time blood reaches capillaries. The pressure wave that traverses ahead of actual movement of blood to the periphery, has higher velocity than the velocity of blood flow (in the aorta, the velocity of pressure wave is 15 times the velocity of blood flow) and is palpable as *arterial pulse* (radial pulse, femoral pulse, etc.). The velocity of transmission of pulse is 3–5 m/s in aorta (as it is more compliant), 7–10 m/s in large arterial branches, 15–35 m/s in small arteries. A typical pressure pulse recording can be obtained from aorta and is proportionate to the pulse pressure, i.e. difference between systolic and diastolic blood pressure, rather than mean pressure. The volume/strength of the pulse depends upon the stoke volume output of the heart and compliance of the arterial tree.

Damping of the pressure pulsations, as the wave traverses towards periphery is due to:

1. Resistance to blood movement in the vessels
2. Compliance of the vessels

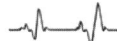

CLINICAL ASPECTS

The following aspects of pulse are clinically studied:
1. Rate
2. Rhythm
3. Volume
4. Character
5. Condition of the vessel wall
6. Radiofemoral delay

A typical pressure pulse recorded from the aorta reveals an upstroke known as *percussion wave,* a downstroke with incisura/dicrotic notch (denoting closure of aortic valves), a *dicrotic wave,* i.e. a reflected wave moving forward, after closure of the aortic valves.

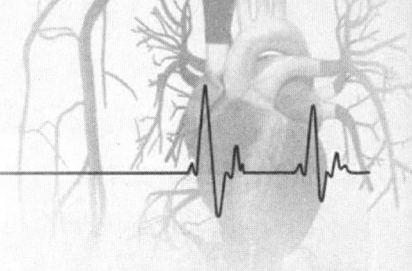

Veins

CENTRAL VENOUS PRESSURE

- Right atrial pressure (RAP) is also known as *central venous pressure.*
- Right atrial pressure is regulated by the balance between ability of blood to flow from peripheral circulation and the ability of heart to pump.
- Normal RAP = 0 mmHg; when the RAP rises to 4 to 6 mmHg, then the peripheral venous pressure rises.
- It can increase to 20–30 mmHg in:
  1. Serious heart failure
  2. After massive transfusion of blood
- Lower limit of –3 to –5 mmHg is reached after:
  1. Haemorrhage or
  2. Increased pumping by the heart.

PERIPHERAL VENOUS PRESSURE

Pressure in the veins is 4–6 mmHg greater than RAP.

Factors influencing Peripheral Venous Pressure

1. *In the abdomen, the veins are compressed by the abdominal organs*: In pregnancy, abdominal tumours, excessive fluid in the abdominal cavity (ascites), etc., the pressure in the peritoneal cavity increases from normal value of 6 mm Hg up to 15–30 mmHg. If the abdominal pressure increases to

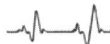

20 mmHg, the pressure in femoral veins also increases to at least 20 mmHg.

2. *In the neck, the veins are compressed by the atmospheric pressure:* Neck veins in the upright position are collapsed due to atmospheric pressure. Thus the pressure in these veins remains zero.

3. *In the arms, compression of veins by the angulation of first rib:* In the arm veins at the level of top of the rib, it is about +6 mmHg, due to compression of subclavian vein as it passes over the rib.

4. *Hydrostatic pressure:* In the vascular system of human being, gravitational pressure is exerted due to the weight of the column of blood in the vessels. In a person who is standing still, the pressure in the feet is 90 mmHg.

5. *In the skull, the veins do not collapse.* There is negative pressure of –10 mmHg in sagittal sinus, due to suction between the top of the skull and base of the skull in the standing position.

VENOUS PUMP

With the movement of the legs, the muscles are tightened and the veins are compressed.

Venous Pump or Muscle Pump

The venous pressure in the feet of a walking adult remains less than 25 mmHg. If one does not move, the value increases to 90 mmHg in 30 seconds. The pressure in the capillaries also increases and fluid leaks into tissue spaces. The legs swell due to leakage of fluid (10–20% of blood volume can be lost while standing still, in the first 15 minutes of standing). The venous valves are positioned in such a way that the blood is squeezed from the compressed veins and flows towards the heart in only one direction. This type of pumping is known as *venous pump or muscle pump.*

The Hydrostatic Level in the Circulatory System

At this level in the circulatory system, the hydrostatic pressure factors, caused by changes in body position of a normal person, do not affect the pressure measurement by more than 1–2 mmHg.

This is the *hydrostatic level in circulatory system.* The level of tricuspid valve is the reference level for pressure measurement.

SPECIFIC RESERVOIRS OF BLOOD

Certain portions of the circulatory system are highly compliant and accommodate large volumes of blood. These are known as *specific blood reservoirs.* They are:
1. Spleen
2. Liver
3. Large abdominal veins
4. Venous plexus under the skin
5. Heart and lungs

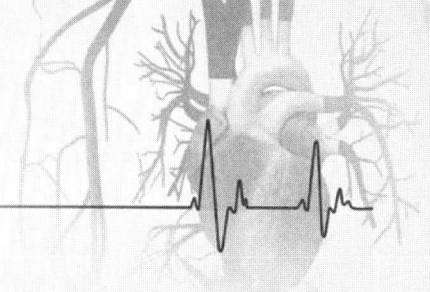

13

Lymphatic System

Lymphatic system carries proteins and large particulate matter from interstitial spaces.

PERMEABILITY OF LYMPHATIC CAPILLARIES

About 90 per cent of the fluid filtered from arterial ends is absorbed through venous ends of capillaries. The remaining 10 per cent, amounting to 2–3 L/day enters through lymphatic capillaries into the venous system.

Substances like proteins are absorbed back through lymphatics. Lymphatics have valves at the tips of terminal lymphatic capillaries. Valves are also present along larger lymphatic vessels, up to the point where they empty into blood circulation.

Lymph Formation

Lymph is derived from interstitial fluid and its composition is same as interstitial fluid. It has protein concentration of 2 gm/dl. Lymph formed in the liver has protein concentration as high as 6 gm/dl. Lymph from intestine has 3–4 gm/dl protein concentration. Thoracic duct lymph, which is a mixture of lymph from all the areas of the body, has 3–5 gm/dl of protein concentration.

In the gastrointestinal tract, absorption of fats and nutrients also occurs through lymphatics. Bacteria can also pass through and are filtered in lymph nodes and destroyed there.

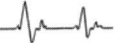

Flow rate of lymph

It is 100 ml/hr through thoracic duct in a resting human and 20 ml/hour through other channels into circulation. Total estimated lymph flow is 120 ml/hr, i.e. 2–3 L/day.

When the interstitial fluid pressure increases to 0 mmHg, the lymph flow increases more than 20 times.

Factors increasing interstitial fluid pressure:
1. ↑ capillary pressure
2. ↓ plasma colloid osmotic pressure
3. ↑ interstitial fluid colloid osmotic pressure
4. ↑ permeability of capillaries.

Lymphatic Pump

Valves are present in large lymphatics and small lymphatics.

Intrinsic pumping: Each segment in between 2 valves, is stretched with lymph and then contracts, emptying the lymph into the next segment. This sort of intrinsic pumping is known as *lymphatic pump*.

In a large lymph vessel like thoracic duct, the lymphatic pump generates pressure as high as 50–100 mmHg.

External factors that cause pumping due to intermittent compression of the lymphatics are:
1. Contraction of surrounding muscles
2. Movement of parts of the body
3. Arterial pulsations
4. Compression of tissues by objects outside the body

Pumping action of lymphatic capillaries: Lymphatic capillary endothelial cells contain contractile actomyosin filaments. Some pumping can be due to rhythmical contraction of lymphatic capillaries. Some pumping in the lymphatic capillaries occurs due to external compression.

↑ increase; ↓ decrease

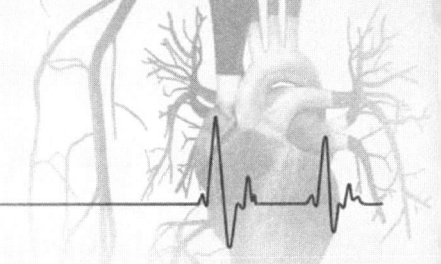

14

Local Control of Blood Flow

SPECIFIC NEEDS OF TISSUES

The tissues control their own blood flow in proportion to their metabolic needs.

The tissues need adequate blood supply to meet their specific requirements like:

1. Supply of O_2, glucose, amino acids, fatty acids, etc.
2. Removal of carbon dioxide and other wastes from tissues
3. Maintenance of proper concentration of other ions in the tissues
4. Transport of various hormones, etc.

The blood flow is maintained at minimum, to supply enough nutrients to the tissues.

BLOOD FLOW OF VARIOUS ORGANS (ml/min/100 gm) (Fig. 14.1)

Blood Flow Control Mechanisms

1. *Acute control*: This occurs within seconds to minutes. It maintains appropriate local tissue blood flow through constriction or dilation of arterioles, meta-arterioles and precapillary sphincters.
2. *Long-term control*: It occurs over a period of days, weeks or months, through an increase or decrease in the actual sizes and numbers of blood vessels supplying the tissues.

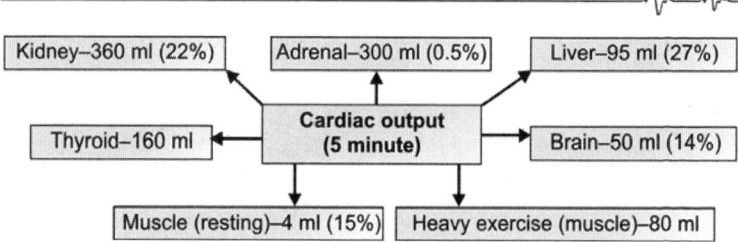

Fig. 14.1: Distribution of cardiac output to various organs

ACUTE CONTROL MECHANISMS OF LOCAL BLOOD FLOW

When the oxygen availability to the tissue decreases or the metabolism of the tissue increases, the blood flow increases accordingly.

1. Metabolism of muscle increases during exercise
2. Availability of oxygen decreases, for example:
   a. At high altitude
   b. Pneumonia
   c. Carbon monoxide poisoning
   d. Cyanide poisoning

Acute control mechanisms can be grouped under the following headings

1. Regulation of blood flow dependent upon tissue metabolism or oxygen/nutrient demand.
2. Special blood flow control mechanisms.
3. Autoregulation.
4. Local factors.
5. Factors secreted by endothelium.

THEORIES FOR ACUTE CONTROL OF BLOOD FLOW

Regulation of Blood Flow, Dependent upon Tissue Metabolism or Oxygen/Nutrient Demand

Two theories are put forward. Both are metabolic control theories:

a. *Vasodilator theory:* Whenever the metabolism of tissues increases, or the tissue demand for oxygen and other nutrients increases, there is proportionate accumulation of the metabolic end products. These are the local vasodilator substances like adenosine, CO_2, lactic acid, adenosine phosphate compounds, histamine, potassium ions and hydrogen ions. These substances diffuse to precapillary sphincters, meta-arterioles and arterioles causing vasodilation, increased blood flow that results in increased supply of oxygen and other nutrients and also washes away the end products of metabolism, e.g. adenosine causing coronary vasodilation.

Drawback of this theory: The measured increase in blood flow, cannot be attributed to any single vasodilator substance, during states of increased tissue metabolic demand or decreased tissue oxygen supply.

b. *Oxygen/nutrient demand theory*: O_2 and other nutrients are required for vascular smooth muscle contraction and in the absence of the same the blood vessels dilate. Besides oxygen, glucose, amino acids, fatty acids, vitamin B substances like thiamine, niacin and riboflavin are required for contraction of vascular smooth muscle.

Increased metabolism → increased utilisation of O_2 → O_2 is required for vascular muscle contraction → blood vessels dilate in the absence of O_2.

Vasomotion

The number of precapillary sphincters that are open at any given time, is proportional to the requirements of the tissues for nutrition. The precapillary sphincters and the meta-arterioles often open and close, several times per minute cyclically and this phenomenon is known as *vasomotion*.

Smooth muscles require O_2 → strength of contraction of the sphincters increases with increase in O_2 concentration → these remain closed.

When O_2 concentration falls → sphincters open.

SPECIAL EXAMPLES OF METABOLIC CONTROL OF BLOOD FLOW

The two other special examples of metabolic control of local blood flow are:
1. Reactive hyperaemia
2. Active hyperaemia

→ leads to

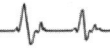

Reactive Hyperaemia

When the blood supply to a tissue is blocked for a few seconds to several hours and then is unblocked, there is 4–7 fold increase in tissue blood flow, that lasts long enough to repay exactly the tissue oxygen deficit that occurred during the period of occlusion. This phenomenon is called *reactive hyperaemia*.

Active Hyperaemia

Blood flow increases in a tissue which is highly active, like an exercising muscle, gland during secretory activity or brain during mental activity. This is known as *active hyperaemia*. Large quantities of vasodilator substances are released and nutrients are utilized. Blood flow in skeletal muscle may increase twenty times during intense exercise.

SPECIAL BLOOD FLOW CONTROL MECHANISMS

Kidneys: Tubuloglomerular Feedback

Decreased glomerular filtration rate (GFR) → Slows the flow rate in loop of Henle → increased reabsorption of Na^+ and Cl^- in the ascending limb of loop of Henle → decrease in the concentration of sodium chloride at the macula densa.

The cells of the macula densa sense the decline in Na^+ and Cl^- in some way and bring about the following effects:

i. Decrease the resistance of the afferent arterioles→ increase in glomerular hydrostatic pressure→GFR increases and returns to normal.

ii. Release of renin from juxtaglomerular cells→ angiotensin I formation→angiotension II formation→ constriction of efferent arterioles→increase in glomerular hydrostatic pressure→GFR returns to normal.

Brain

In addition to control of blood flow by tissue O_2 concentration, an increase in the concentration of carbon dioxide and hydrogen ions, dilates the cerebral blood vessels → increase in cerebral blood flow → rapid washout of excess CO_2 and hydrogen ions.

→ leads to

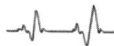

AUTOREGULATION OF BLOOD FLOW

When there is an acute increase in arterial pressure, there is proportionate increase in blood flow. Despite the increased arterial pressure, the tissues tend to regulate their own blood flow. In the pressure range of 70 to 175 mmHg, when the arterial pressure increases one and half times, the blood flow increases only by 30 per cent. This is known as *autoregulation*.

Theories put forward for autoregulation

1. Metabolic theory
2. Myogenic theory

Metabolic Theory

Increased arterial pressure (mmHg) → excess blood flow → excess O_2 and other nutrients supplied to the tissues → these nutrients cause blood vessels to constrict and the flow returns to nearly normal despite increased pressure.

Myogenic Theory

Sudden stretch of small blood vessels → smooth muscle of the vessel wall contracts → reduces blood flow nearly back to normal.

At low pressures → degree of stretch of the vessel is less → smooth muscle relaxes → flow increases.

The role played by the vascular smooth muscle in the myogenic theory of autoregulation is doubtful as the increase in pressure causes increased contraction of the vascular smooth muscle → increase in total peripheral resistance (TPR) → further increase in pressure → further contraction will lead to tremendous increase in arterial pressure all over the body.

The autoregulation protects the capillaries from damage, when blood pressure rises to excessively high values.

LOCAL FACTORS

Local Vasodilator Substances

Justify both the metabolic theories of local blood flow control mechanisms, i.e. vasodilator theory and O_2/nutrient demand theory:

→ leads to

1. $\downarrow O_2$, pH
2. $\uparrow pCO_2$
3. $\uparrow$ temperature
4. $\uparrow K^+$, end products of metabolism, $\uparrow Mg^{++}$, $\uparrow Na^+$
5. Acetate and citrate, $\uparrow H^+$
6. Histamine, adenosine

Local Vasoconstrictors

1. $\uparrow O_2$
2. Serotonin
3. $\downarrow$ temperature
4. $\downarrow H^+$
5. $\uparrow Ca^{++}$

Increase in pCO_2 causes moderate vasodilation in tissues and marked vasodilation in the brain. However, through vasomotor centre, it exerts powerful vasoconstrictor effect.

SUBSTANCES SECRETED BY ENDOTHELIUM

Vasodilators

Endothelium derived relaxing factor (EDRF, nitric oxide), prostacyclin.

Vasoconstrictors

Endothelin, thromboxane A_2

Endothelium Derived Relaxing Factor (EDRF, Nitric Oxide, NO)

In 1998, RF Furchgott, F Murad and LJ Ignarro got the Nobel Prize for discovery of NO. Whenever the microvascular blood flow increases, endothelial cells lining the arterioles and small arteries synthesize substances, that cause increase in the dimension of larger blood vessels upstream. The most important of these is EDRF (nitric oxide).

NO is synthesised from arginine and its synthesis is catalysed by an enzyme, NOS (nitric oxide synthase).

$\downarrow$ decrease; $\uparrow$ increase

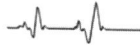

Three Isoforms of Nitric Oxide Synthase

- NOS 1: Found in nervous system
- NOS 2: Found in macrophages and other immune cells
- NOS 3: Found in endothelial cells

Nitric oxide has a half life of only 6 seconds. It is a gas and acts in a paracrine fashion. NOS 1 and NOS 3 are activated by agents that increase intracellular Ca^{++} concentration (e.g. vasodilators like acetylcholine and bradykinin). NOS 2 in immune cells is activated by cytokines.

Multiple Stimuli Cause Release of Nitric Oxide

1. Acetylcholine
2. Bradykinin, VIP, substance P, ATP and histamine via H_1 receptors
3. Various vasoconstrictors act on vascular endothelium, to release NO simultaneously.
4. Products of platelet aggregation also cause release of NO. It helps to keep blood vessels with an intact endothelium patent.

Physiological Effects of NO

1. Tonic release of NO is required for maintenance of normal blood pressure. NO deficiency can cause clinical hypertension.
2. NO is responsible for penile erection.
3. NO is present in brain. It is a gas and diffuses easily and binds to guanylyl cyclase. It may be the signal by which postsynaptic neurons communicate with presynaptic endings, in *long-term potentiation* and *long-term depression*.
4. It is important for the cytotoxic activity of macrophages and their ability to kill cancer cells.
5. In gastrointestinal tract, it is a major dilator of smooth muscle.

Prostacyclin and Thromboxane A_2

Prostacyclin is produced by endothelial cells and thromboxane A_2 is produced by platelets from arachidonic acid via cyclo-oxygenase pathway.

Thromboxane A_2 causes platelet aggregation and vasoconstriction prostacyclin: Inhibits platelet aggregation and causes vasodilation

The drug aspirin causes irreversible inhibition of cyclo-oxygenase→↑production of both thromboxane A_2 and prostacyclin.

However, endothelial cells produce new cyclo-oxygenase but platelets cannot synthesise this. Hence, prostacyclin is still formed, inhibiting platelet aggregation and causing vasodilation.

Endothelins

Endothelin-1(ET-1) is the most potent vasoconstrictor agent. ET-1, ET-2 and ET-3 are encoded by different genes.

- *Endothelin-1:* Found in brain, kidneys and endothelial cells
- *Endothelin-2:* Primarily in kidneys and intestine
- *Endothelin-3:* Is present in blood and in high concentration in the brain. It is also found in the kidneys and GI tract.

Endothelins are found abundantly in the brain and in early life are produced by both astrocytes and neurons. They are found in dorsal root ganglia, ventral horn cells, the hypothalamus and cerebellar Purkinje cells. They regulate transport across blood–brain barrier.

Endothelin-1

Endothelin-1 is primarily a local paracrine regulator of vascular tone. Big endothelin-1 and endothelin-1 are both present in the circulation. The product of endothelin-1 gene is processed to 39 amino acid prohormone, big endothelin-1. The prohormone is cleaved by endothelin converting enzyme. Small amounts of big endothelin-1 and endothelin-1 are secreted into the blood, but mostly into the media of blood vessels and act in a paracrine manner.

- Two different endothelin receptors have been cloned. They are coupled to phospholipase C via G proteins.
- ET_A *receptor:* Specific to endothelin-1, is found in many tissues and mediates vasoconstriction.

→ leads to; ↑ increase

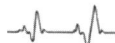

- ET_B *receptor:* Binds to all three endothelins and is coupled to G_i. It may mediate vasodilation.

Principal Actions

1. Contraction of vascular smooth muscle, intense vasoconstriction of coronary arteries
2. Positive inotropic and positive chronotropic effects on myocardium
3. Causes increase in plasma levels of ANP, renin, aldosterone and catecholamines. Modulates synaptic transmission
4. Decreases GFR, renal blood flow and glomerular ultrafiltration coefficient and increases renal vascular resistance
5. Causes bronchoconstriction
6. Enhances gluconeogenesis
7. Regulates gastrointestinal blood flow

LONG-TERM LOCAL BLOOD FLOW REGULATION

If the tissue becomes chronically overactive → requires chronically increased quantities of nutrients › blood supply increases.

Change in tissue vascularity: If the arterial pressure falls to 60 mmHg and remains at this level for many weeks, the physical structural sizes of the vessels and even the number of vessels in the tissue increases. If metabolism of a tissue increases over a prolonged period, vascularity increases. Conversely, if the arterial pressure increases, the number and sizes of vessels decrease.

This growth of new vessels or reconstruction of vasculature occurs quickly within days in neonates and new tissue, but may take even months or years in elderly persons or old tissue. In younger tissues, the vascularity exactly matches the needs of the tissue for blood flow. In older tissues, vascularity frequently lags far behind the need of the tissues.

Role of O_2: O_2 is important for acute control of local blood flow and also for long-term control. At high altitude, increase in vascularity occurs in animals.

→ leads to

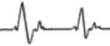

ANGIOGENESIS AND ANGIOGENIC FACTORS

Angiogenesis

It is defined as the growth of new blood vessels in response to the presence of angiogenic factors released from:

1. Ischaemic tissues
2. Tissues that are growing rapidly
3. Tissues that have excessively high metabolic rates

Angiogenic Factors

1. Endothelial cell growth factor (ECGF)
2. Fibroblast growth factor (FGF)
3. Angiogenin (isolated from tumours or from other tissues that have inadequate blood supply)

New vessel formation from existing small vessels: Dissolution of basement membrane of the endothelial cells → rapid reproduction of new endothelial cells, that stream out of the vessel wall in the form of cords, directed towards the source of angiogenic factors → cells in a particular cord divide and eventually fold into a tube that connects with another tube budding from another donor vessel → forms capillary loop → blood begins to flow → if flow is great, smooth muscle cells invade the wall → new vessels grow into arterioles or even larger arteries.

COLLATERAL CIRCULATION

When an artery or a vein is blocked, new vascular channel develops around the blockage and dilation of the vessel, that already connects the vessel above the block and below the block, occurs.

With initial opening of collateral vessels, blood supply/flow is usually still less than one-fourth needed to supply tissue needs. With further opening, within a day, 50 per cent of tissue needs are fulfilled. Then within a few days, almost all tissue needs are met. Under resting conditions, blood flow remains normal. However, during strenuous tissue activity that requires maximal blood flow, the tissue collateral flow is unable to meet the tissue demands.

→ leads to

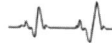

SYSTEMIC VASODILATORS AND VASOCONSTRICTORS

Systemic Vasodilators

1. Adenosine (also local), ANP and histamine via H_2 receptor produce relaxation of vascular smooth muscle, that is independent of endothelium.
2. Acetylcholine, bradykinin, VIP, substance P, some systemic polypeptides and histamine via H_1 receptor act via endothelium and cause vasodilation.
3. Serotonin can have both vasoconstrictor and vasodilatory effects.

Systemic Vasoconstrictors

Circulating vasoconstrictor hormones include vasopressin, norepinephrine, epinephrine and angiotensin II. Various vasoconstrictors act directly on vascular smooth muscle and also simultaneously cause the release of NO.

Kinins (Fig. 14.2)

The decapeptide lysylbradykinin, also known as kalidin and the nonapeptide bradykinin are two vasodilator peptides found in the body.

- Lysylbradykinin is converted to bradykinin by aminopeptidase. Biological activities of both components are similar.
- High molecular weight (HMW) kininogen and low molecular weight (LMW) kininogen are produced by alternative splicing of a single gene located on chromosome 3. Active plasma kallikrein converts HMW kininogen to bradykinin. Tissue kallikrein converts HMW and LMW kininogen to lysylbradykinin.
- Kininase I and kininase II inactivate both peptides. Kininase II is same as angiotensin-converting enzyme.

There are two bradykinin receptors, B_1 and B_2. Both are serpentine receptors coupled to G-proteins.

Physiological Actions

1. They are tissue hormones. Small amounts are found in blood.
2. They cause contraction of visceral smooth muscle.

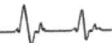

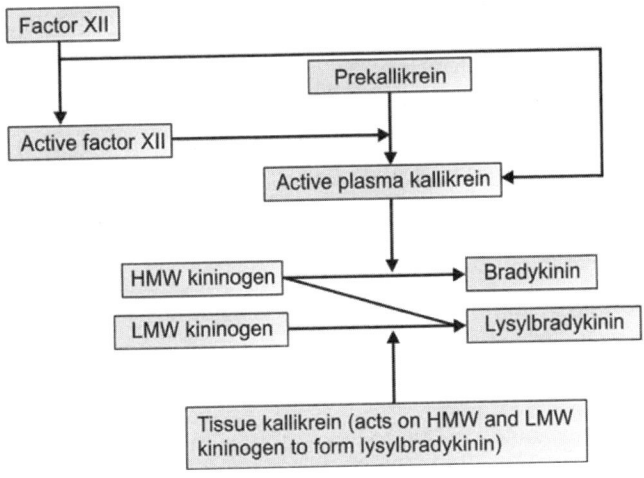

Fig. 14.2: Formation of bradykinin and lysylbradykinin

3. They relax vascular smooth muscle via NO and decrease blood pressure.
4. They increase blood flow in active tissues.
5. They increase capillary permeability, attract leucocytes and cause pain upon injection under skin.
6. They are formed during active secretion in sweat glands, salivary glands and exocrine portion of pancreas.

Atrial Natriuretic Peptide (ANP)

ANP has 28 amino acid residues.

Brain Natriuretic Peptide (BNP)

It was isolated from porcine brain. It is present in human brain, blood and heart.

C-Type Natriuretic Peptide (CNP)

It is present in human brain, kidneys, pituitary, vascular endothelial cells.

Secretion and Metabolism

Concentration of ANP in plasma is 5 mol/ml in normal humans ingesting moderate amounts of sodium. Muscle cells in atria have secretory granules for ANP.

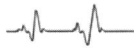

- ANP secretion increases when ECF volume is increased by infusion of isotonic saline or ingestion of high sodium diet.
- Immersion in water up to neck causes increase in central venous pressure, causing increase in atrial pressure and secretion of ANP.

Physiological Actions of ANP

1. Causes natriuresis:
   a. By binding to ANP receptors on mesangial cells in the glomeruli, causes relaxation of the cells and increases the effective surface area available for filtration, or
   b. By acting on tubules, promotes sodium excretion and inhibits Na^+ reabsorption.
2. ANP lowers blood pressure.
3. Decreases responsiveness of vascular smooth muscle to many vasoconstrictor substances.
4. Decreases the responsiveness of zona glomerulosa to stimuli, that increase the aldosterone secretion and inhibits secretion of vasopressin.
5. Inhibits renin secretion and lowers circulating angiotensin II levels. All the three, i.e. ANP, BNP and CNP, exert their effects through cyclic-GMP.

ANP Receptors

There are three different types of receptors.

NPR-A, NPR-B and NPR-C: They span the cell membrane and have cytoplasmic domains that are guanylyl cyclases. ANP has greatest affinity for NPR-A receptors. CNP has greatest affinity for NPR-B receptors. NPR-C combines all three. It has a truncated cytoplasmic domain that acts via G proteins to activate phospholipase C and inhibits adenylyl cyclase.

Microcirculation

DEFINITION

It is defined as the circulation of blood through the arterioles, the meta-arterioles, the capillaries and venules, the smallest vessels of the body.

Arterioles

Diameter of the arterioles is 20–50 μm. The arterioles consist of thick smooth muscle layer and are sites of maximum resistance to blood flow. Hence the pressure drops across them is maximum.

Meta-arterioles

The meta-arterioles arise from the arterioles, are 10–15 μm in diameter, have smooth muscle fibres encircling the vessel at intermittent points and open into the capillaries. At the point where the meta-arteriole opens into the capillary, it is surrounded by a ring of smooth muscle fibres, known as *precapillary sphincter*.

Flow of blood is intermittent, on and off, every few seconds or minutes, due to contraction of smooth muscle fibres of meta-arterioles and precapillary sphincters. This is known as *vasomotion*.

Capillaries

The capillaries are single layer of highly permeable endothelial cells. Exchange of nutrients and cellular wastes occurs here. There are about ten billion capillaries and the total surface area is 500 to 700 square meters. Single functional tissue cell is about 20 to 30 μm away from the capillary. Thickness of the capillary wall is 0.5 μm and is composed of basement membrane on outside and endothelial cell layer inside. Diameter of the capillaries is 5–9 μm. There are pores in the capillaries, which are intercellular clefts of 6–7 nm diameter. The pores vary in size in different tissues. In brain, these are tight junctions. In liver, these are large pores, through which almost all dissolved substances including plasma proteins pass. In the kidneys, there are fenestrae in the middle of endothelial cells, through which ionic substances pass.

EXCHANGE OF WATER AND NUTRIENTS

Diffusion

Water and dissolved particles diffuse as a result of thermal motion of water molecules and dissolved substances. Lipid-soluble substances like O_2 and CO_2 can diffuse easily through the entire length of capillary.

However, water, sodium, chloride ions and glucose, pass through intercellular clefts only. The velocity of thermal molecular motion in the clefts is so great that the water of the plasma exchanges with water of interstitial fluid at least 80 times, before plasma leaves the other end of the capillary. Permeability varies with the molecular size and water has highest permeability and albumin the least.

The net rate of diffusion of a substance through any membrane is proportionate to the concentration difference between the two sides of the membrane. Very small concentration difference is required for the substances to diffuse through the pores.

INTERSTITIAL FLUID

Interstitium

The interstitium has
1. *Collagen fibre bundles*: That are extremely strong and provide tensile strength.
2. *Proteoglycan filaments*: That are delicate, form mat of very fine reticular filaments.

Fluid in interstitium is formed by filtration and diffusion from capillaries. It contains same constituents as plasma except lower concentration of proteins. Interstitial fluid is entrapped in minute spaces among proteoglycan filaments. The proteoglycan filaments and the fluid entrapped within them have characteristics of a gel and is called *tissue gel*. There are rivulets of free fluid in the interstitium.

Starling Forces

Four primary forces determine fluid movement through capillary membrane:

1. *The capillary pressure (Pc):* It tends to force fluid outward through the capillary membrane.
2. *The interstitial fluid pressure (Pif):* When Pif is positive, fluid moves inward through the capillary membrane and when Pif is negative, fluid moves outward.
3. *The plasma colloid osmotic pressure (πp):* Due to osmotic pressure exerted by the plasma proteins, fluid moves inward through the capillary membrane.
4. *The interstitial fluid colloid osmotic pressure (πif):* Due to osmotic pressure of the proteins in the interstitium, fluid moves outward through the capillary membrane.

Capillary Pressure

The capillary pressure can be determined by direct cannulation. It is 30–40 mmHg at the arterial ends and 10–15 mmHg at the venous ends.

By indirect functional measurement of capillary pressure through isogravimetric method, it is 17.3 mmHg.

Interstitial Fluid Pressure

It can be measured by direct cannulation of the tissues with a micropipette, through implanted perforated capsules or through cotton wick inserted into the tissue. It is −1 to −3 mmHg.

Interstitial fluid pressure in tightly encased tissues: It is highly positive, ranging from +4 to +13 mmHg, as the encasements exert pressure on the tissues, e.g. cranial vault around the brain, fibrous capsules around the kidney, etc.

Plasma Colloid Osmotic Pressure

Proteins do not diffuse readily through the capillary membrane.

Proteins are present in the following concentrations:
- 7.3 gm/dl in plasma
- 2–3 gm/dl in interstitial fluid

Proteins exert colloid osmotic pressure or oncotic pressure. The osmotic pressure that results at the cell membrane is called total osmotic pressure, to distinguish it from colloid osmotic pressure. Colloid osmotic pressure of the human plasma averages about 28 mmHg, 19 mmHg is due to dissolved proteins and 9 mmHg is exerted by cations (Donnan effect).

Reflection coefficient: When protein molecules are unable to pass through pores, they are reflected and osmotic pressure is a product of this reflection process. When all the protein molecules are reflected, the reflection coefficient is 1.0 and when none, it is zero. The brain and muscle have reflection coefficient as 1 and the liver zero. Osmotic pressure is determined by the mass of the protein molecules. Albumin contributes to 80% of the colloid osmotic pressure, globulin 20% and fibrinogen nil.

Interstitial Fluid Colloid Osmotic Pressure

The concentration of proteins, that do leak through the pores is 3 gm/dl in 12 litres of interstitial fluid. The average colloid osmotic pressure for this concentration of proteins is 8 mmHg, when the reflection coefficient is one.

Starling Equilibrium (Fig. 15.1)

The fluid that is filtered through the arterial end of the capillaries is reabsorbed through the venous ends.

EH Starling pointed out that a state of near equilibrium exists at capillary membrane, as the amount of fluid filtered outwards from arterial ends of capillaries, is exactly same as the amount of fluid returning to circulation by absorption through venous capillaries. The rest of the fluid returns by way of lymphatics (1/10th of the filtered fluid).

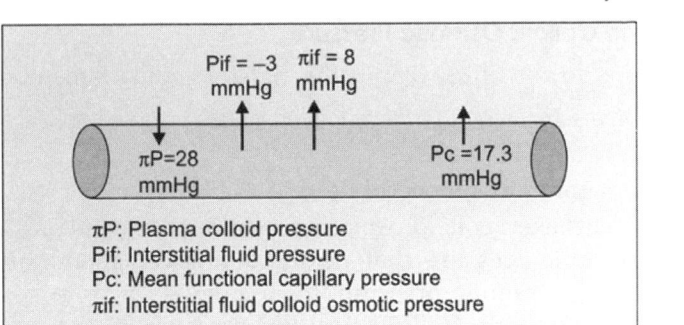

Fig. 15.1: Starling equilibrium for capillary exchange

The Starling forces are calculated in the following manner:

Mean forces tending to move fluid outward	In mmHg
Mean capillary pressure	17.3
Negative interstitial fluid pressure	3.0
Interstitial fluid colloid osmotic pressure	8.0
Total outward force	28.3
Mean forces tending to move fluid inward	
Plasma colloid osmotic pressure	28.0
Net outward force, tending to move fluid out	0.3 mmHg

Filtration coefficient: There is a net imbalance of forces at capillary membrane of 0.3 mmHg. This causes net rate of fluid filtration in the entire body of 2 ml/min. It turns out to be 6.67 ml/min/mmHg for the entire body. This is called the *filtration coefficient.*

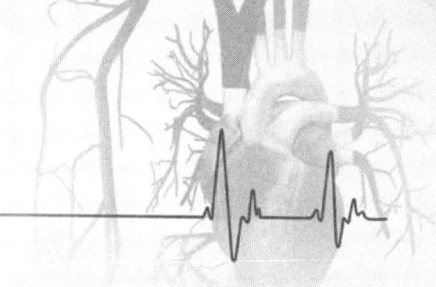

16

Circulatory Shock

DEFINITION

Circulatory shock is defined as generalised inadequacy of blood flow throughout the body, resulting in less delivery of O_2 and other nutrients to the tissues and inadequate removal of cellular wastes from the body tissues, causing damage to them. Various causes of circulatory shock are given in Fig. 16.1.

Stages of Shock

1. *Non-progressive stage (compensated stage):* Normal circulatory compensatory mechanisms of the body come into play. Full recovery occurs without help from interventional therapy.
2. *Progressive stage:* Becomes steadily worse until death. Up to certain limit (both duration of shock and severity), interventional therapy can still be helpful.
3. *Irreversible stage:* Beyond a critical stage, all forms of known therapy are inadequate.

A classical experiment is conducted to demonstrate the progression of circulatory shock through various stages, in which a dog is bled rapidly so that the arterial pressure decreased to different levels (*haemorrhagic shock*). During this experiment, it was observed that there is a critical level of arterial pressure, beyond which if the blood volume is further reduced, the negative feedback mechanisms fail to operate and shock breeds more shock. At this stage, the progressive stage sets in and a number of positive feedback mechanisms, which are detrimental to the body, start operating.

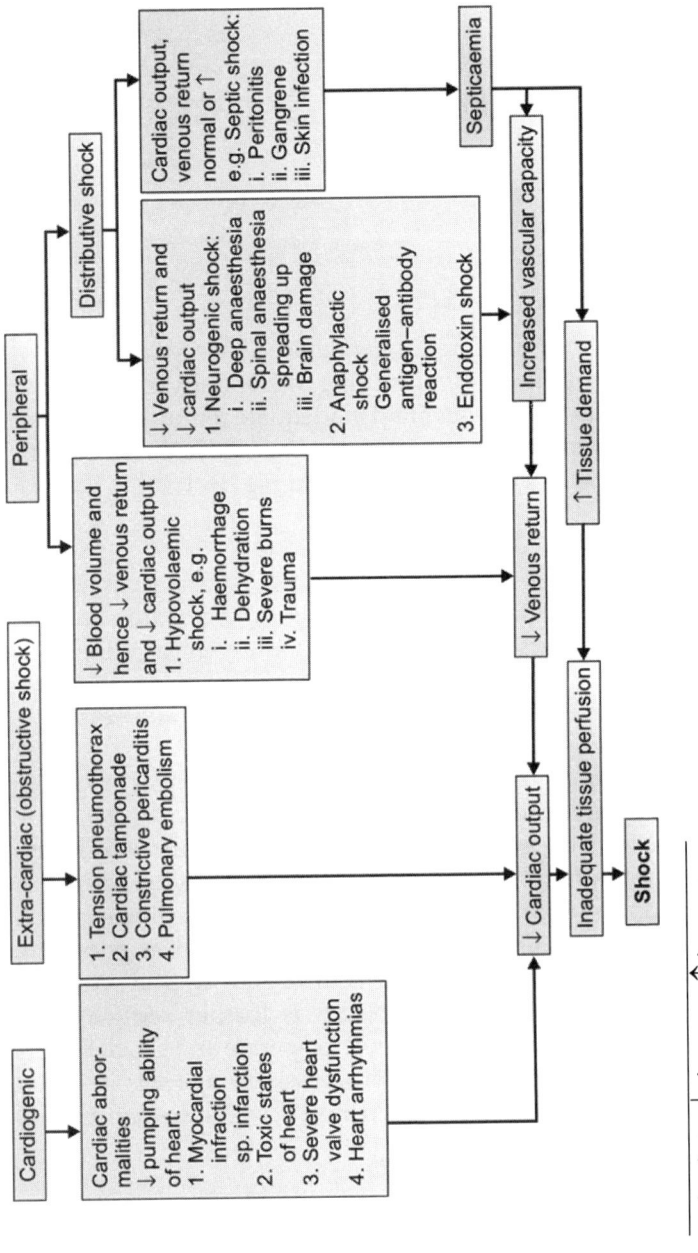

Fig. 16.1: Classification of circulatory shock

→ leads to; ↓ decrease; ↑ increase

Haemorrhagic shock is the most common cause of hypovolaemic shock. The arterial pressure or cardiac output remain normal when 10 per cent of total blood volume is removed. In the absence of sympathetic reflexes, only 15–20 per cent of blood volume, over a period of 30 minutes can be removed. Whereas with intact reflexes, 30–40 per cent loss of blood volume can be sustained. The cardiac output and arterial pressure fall to zero when 35–45 per cent of total blood volume has been removed. Cardiac output declines first. Sympathetic reflexes are geared more for maintaining arterial pressure.

Sympathetic Reflex Compensatory Mechanisms

1. Baroreceptors and low pressure vascular stretch receptors in the thorax elicit powerful sympathetic reflexes → sympathetic vasoconstrictor system is stimulated.
   a. Arterioles constrict throughout the body→↑ in total peripheral resistance (TPR)
   b. Veins and venous reservoirs constrict → adequate venous return (VR), despite ↓ blood volume
   c. Increased heart activity: Heat rate increases from 72 to 170–200 beats/min.
2. Coronary and cerebral blood flow are protected. Auto-regulation is most powerful in both these vascular beds. The sympathetic vasoconstrictor innervation is minimal. Thus, sympathetic stimulation does not cause powerful vasoconstriction in both these beds. Blood flow is maintained at normal levels as long as arterial pressure does not fall ↓70 mmHg.
3. In organs like kidneys, there is profound vasoconstriction of precapillary sphincters and venules with prolonged sympathetic stimulation, causing renal shutdown.

Non-progressive Stage (Fig. 16.2)

If shock is not severe enough to cause its own progression, *non-progressive or compensated shock* occurs. At this stage, negative feedback circulatory compensatory mechanisms operate.

→ leads to; ↓ decrease; ↑ increase

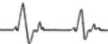

Compensatory Mechanisms

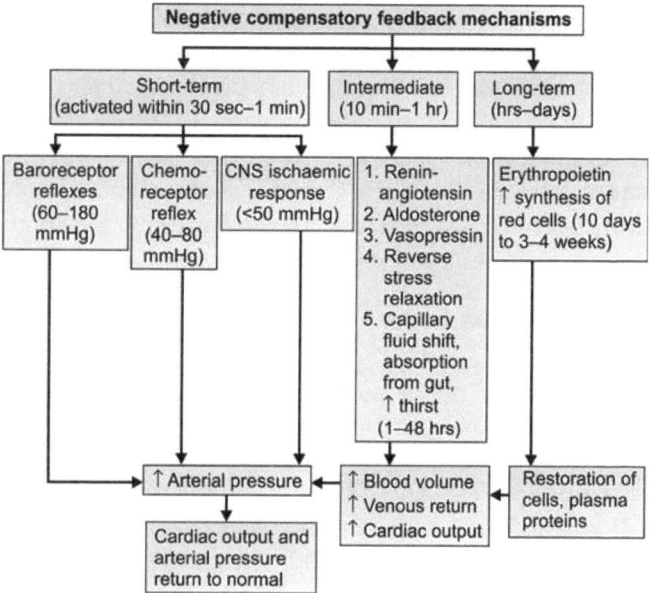

Fig. 16.2: Non-progressive stage of shock showing the negative compensatory feedback mechanisms (↑ increase)

Progressive Stage

Once shock has become severe and reached a critical stage and lasts longer at this stage, the structures of the circulatory system begin to deteriorate and positive feedback mechanisms start operating, leading to progressive shock.

Positive Feedback Mechanisms (Fig. 16.3)

Positive feedback mechanisms do not always lead to a vicious circle. In mild degrees of shock, the negative feedback mechanisms overcome the positive feedback mechanisms. The arterial pressure may be misleading sometimes, as the sympathetic nervous reflexes are tuned to maintain arterial pressure normal. However, with severe blood loss, both arterial pressure and cardiac output decrease. Once circulatory

1. Cardiac failure

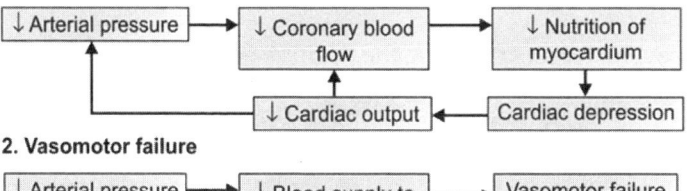

2. Vasomotor failure

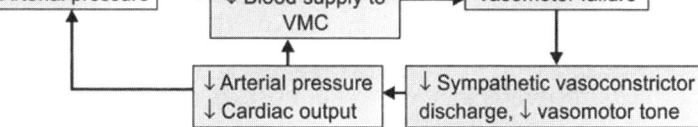

3. Peripheral circulatory failure

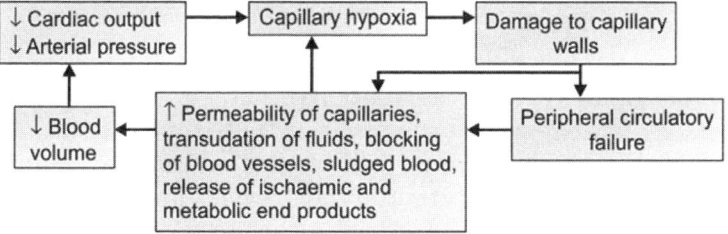

4. Peripheral circulatory failure and cardiac failure

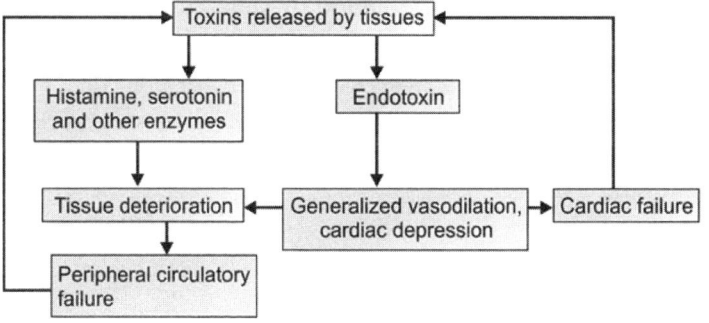

5. Multi-organ failure

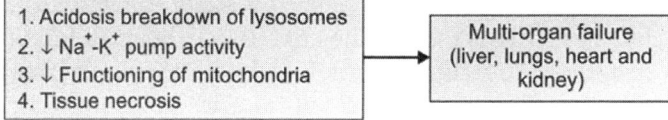

Fig. 16.3: Progressive stage (1–5) of shock showing various positive feedback loops that are detrimental to the body (↑ increase; ↓ decrease)

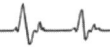

shock reaches a critical state of severity, shock itself breeds more shock.

In severe degrees of shock, the positive feedback mechanisms become more and more powerful → rapid deterioration of circulation → all negative feedback systems acting together cannot return the cardiac output to normal. Thus inadequate blood supply leads to decrease in cardiac output, decrease in tissue perfusion, more shock and death ultimately.

It is a vicious circle and leads to irreversible shock. If the cardiac output falls to one-third of normal, one can survive for a few hours only.

Irreversible Shock

After shock has progressed to a certain stage, transfusion or any other type of interventional therapy cannot save a person's life. Irreversible shock sets in. With blood transfusion, rarely the arterial pressure and cardiac output may return to normal. Beyond certain point, even normal cardiac output cannot reverse the effects of severe shock because of extensive cellular damage, release of destructive enzymes into body fluids, acidosis and depletion of high energy phosphate reserves.

The physiological basis of irreversible shock is the following:

ATP → ADP → AMP → adenosine → comes out of cells, enters circulation → converted to uric acid → uric acid cannot re-enter the cells.

GENERAL FEATURES

1. *Muscle weakness:* Severe muscle weakness and fatigue result, with attempt to use.
2. *Depressed mental function: In early stages:* Mental haziness occurs though the patient may be conscious. This progresses to state of stupor. In the last stages, subconscious functions like vasomotor failure and respiratory failure occur.

→ leads to next step

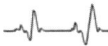

3. *Reduced renal function and renal deterioration:*
   a. *Early stages:* Even slight ↓ in cardiac output and arterial pressure, occurring in the early stages of shock → ↓ glomerular pressure below the critical level required for filtration → urine output greatly diminished or even abolished.
   b. *Late stages:* Tubular epithelial cells having high metabolic rate deteriorate, leading to severe tubular necrosis → tubular cell death → sloughing and blocking of tubules → once this occurs, even if the person survives → kidney damage leads to renal shutdown, with death occurring eventually.

DIFFERENT TYPES OF SHOCK

Specific Clinical Features and their Physiological Basis

1. **Hypovolaemic shock caused by haemorrhage (cold shock):**
   Due to maximum sympathetic discharge:
   i. The skin is pale, cold, cyanotic
   ii. Tachycardia, thin thready pulse
   iii. ↑ Respiratory rate and force
   iv. Oliguria
   v. Restlessness, apprehension
2. **Hypovolaemic shock caused by plasma loss/fluid loss:**
   i. *Burns:* Due to increased blood viscosity, there is sluggishness of blood flow, added on to the decrease in blood volume.
   ii. Intestinal obstruction → blocking of venous blood flow→↑ intestinal capillary pressure → leakage of fluid into the intestinal wall and lumen→ ↓in total plasma protein and plasma volume.
   iii. *Dehydration:* ↓ Blood volume due to loss of fluid.
3. **Hypovolaemic shock caused by trauma/accident:** Due to trauma/accident, there can be contusions of the body without hemorrhage, causing damage to capillaries, leading to excessive loss of plasma into tissues. Extreme pain can

---

→ leads to next step; ↓ decrease; ↑ increase

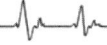

cause inhibition of vasomotor centre leading to ↓ sympathetic discharge.

4. **Warm shock (distributive shock):** *Skin is warm due to vasodilation:*
   a. Neurogenic shock
   b. Anaphylactic shock
   c. Septic shock

   a. *Neurogenic shock:* Sudden loss of vasomotor tone throughout the body →massive dilatation of the veins occurs → ↓ venous return due to ↑ in vascular capacity→↓ mean systemic filling pressure (Psf) → venous pooling

   b. *Anaphylactic shock:* Antigen–antibody reaction leading to activation of basophils in blood and mast cells in pericapillary tissues, resulting in release of histamine or histamine-like substances which cause:
      i. ↑ Vascular capacity due to venous dilatation
      ii. Dilatation of arterioles resulting in ↓ arterial pressure
      iii. ↑ Capillary permeability with rapid loss of fluid and protein into tissue spaces leading to great reduction in venous return. Person dies within minutes.

   c. *Septic shock (classically known as blood poisoning):* Widely disseminated bacterial infection spreads from one tissue to another, causing widespread infection and damage.

   Different infections of different body tissues lead to different effects. This is extremely important type of shock, as this most frequently causes death even in a modern hospital, besides the cardiogenic shock.
      i. High fever, increased metabolic rate
      ii. Marked vasodilation throughout the body
      iii. Due to release of toxins, there is high rate of metabolism and vasodilation in the infected and other tissues giving rise to high cardiac output.
      iv. Sludged blood: There is red cell agglutination in response to degenerating tissue products, blockage of small vessels, decreasing the flow of blood, resulting in *sludged blood.*

→ leads to, next step; ↓ decrease; ↑ increase

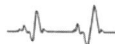

v. As a consequence to development of microclots in the blood vessels resulting in disseminated intravascular coagulation, the clotting factors are used up and haemorrhages occur in many tissues.

In the early stages, there are only signs of bacterial infection. In the later stages, the circulatory system gets involved and the shock progression occurs like any other type of shock.

5. **Endotoxin shock:** It is a special type of septic shock. It frequently occurs when a large segment of gut becomes strangulated and loses most of its blood supply. Gut becomes gangrenous and gram-negative bacteria in the gut multiply (colon bacilli). They release endotoxin.

Endotoxin

1. Decreases myocardial contractility
2. Also causes an effect similar to anaphylaxis

PHYSIOLOGY OF TREATMENT

1. Raising the foot end of the patient's bed by 1', promotes the venous return and cardiac output and improves the blood supply to brain, thus preserving the vital centres. This is especially important in haemorrhagic and neurogenic shock, when blood pressure is low.

2. *Room temperature:* The skin of the patients with shock is cold due to enhanced sympathetic discharge. The sympathetic discharge is maximal in hypovolaemic shock. Any attempt to cover the patient with blankets/keep the person warm will cause abolition of sympathetic discharge and further deterioration of the body compensatory mechanisms.

3. Oxygen therapy may have some beneficial effects

4. Glucocorticoids are useful in advanced stages of shock. They stabilise lysosomal membranes. They increase strength of contraction of the heart and help in the metabolism of glucose.

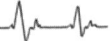

Specific Therapy for Different Types of Shock

Hypovolaemic Shock

a. *Haemorrhagic shock:* Transfusion of whole blood/plasma/plasma expanders like dextran

b. *Burns/intestinal obstruction, etc:* A plasma substitute may be given like dextran. The plasma substitute should fulfill the following requirements:

   i. It should remain in circulation.
   ii. It should be non-toxic.
   iii. Contains appropriate electrolytes.
   iv. Should contain some substances that have a large molecular size, to exert colloidal osmotic pressure.

c. *Dehydration:* Intravenous infusion of electrolyte solution

Neurogenic and Anaphylactic Shock

Sympathomimetic drugs are useful. Norepinephrine, epinephrine and some long-acting drugs can be given.

In anaphylactic shock, life-saving drugs like glucocorticoids counter the effect of histamine.

Septic Shock

Antibiotics should be given.

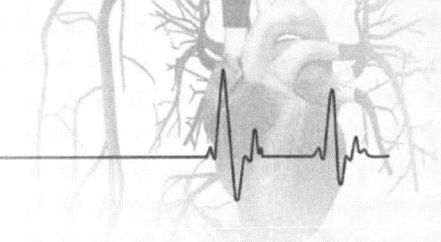

Coronary Circulation

ANATOMICAL ASPECTS

Coronary flow at rest in humans is about 250 ml/min. At rest, heart extracts 70–80 per cent of O_2 from each unit of blood delivered to it. Blood flow increases when metabolism increases. The right and the left coronary arteries arise from the sinuses behind the two cusps of the aortic valve, at the root of the aorta.

In 50 per cent persons, the right coronary artery has greater flow. The left coronary artery has greater flow in 20 per cent persons. Both the coronary arteries have equal flow in 30 per cent individuals. The venous drainage of the heart is through coronary sinus and anterior cardiac veins into right atrium.

Arteriosinusoidal Vessels

They directly open into heart chambers. They are sinusoidal, capillary-like vessels, that connect arterioles to heart chambers.

Thebesian Veins

Connect capillaries to heart chambers.

Arterioluminal Vessels

They are small arteries, draining directly into the chambers. Around the mouths of the great veins, there are a few anastomoses between coronary arterioles and extracardiac arterioles.

135

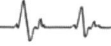

The rate of coronary blood flow is influenced by pressure changes in aorta and by chemical and neural factors.

PRESSURE GRADIENTS AND FLOW (Table 17.1)

When the heart contracts, it compresses the blood vessels. During systole, the pressure inside the left ventricle is slightly higher than in the aorta. The flow is compromised in the subendocardial portions of the left ventricle during systole. However, some flow occurs throughout cardiac cycle in the superficial myocardial layers of the left ventricle. As the flow is compromised during systole, the subendocardial portions of the left ventricle are more prone to ischaemic damage. The pressure gradient between aorta and right ventricle and aorta and atria, is larger during systole. Consequently, coronary flow is not compromised during systole. In aortic stenosis, coronary flow is compromised.

Table 17.1: Pressure (mmHg) changes during systole and diastole

	Systole	Diastole
Pressure in aorta	120	80
Pressure in left ventricle	121	0
Pressure in right ventricle	25	0
Pressure differential between aorta and left ventricle	–1	80
Aorta and right ventricle	95	80

REGULATORY FACTORS

Coronary blood flow decreases if there is decrease in effective coronary perfusion pressure, e.g. in congestive heart failure. Coronary flow also decreases when aortic diastolic pressure is low and in aortic stenosis when the left ventricular pressure during systole is high.

Chemical

O_2 lack, ↑ local concentrations of CO_2, H^+, K^+, lactate, prostaglandins, adenine nucleotides and adenosine cause

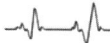

increase in coronary blood flow. Asphyxia, hypoxia increase coronary blood flow 2–3 times.

Neural

1. α-adrenergic receptors of the coronary arterioles mediate vasoconstriction
2. β-adrenergic receptors mediate vasodilation

However, when arterial pressure falls, activity in noradrenergic nerves to the heart and injections of norepinephrine cause vasodilation. This is secondary to the increased activity of the heart by norepinephrine as vasodilator metabolites are produced in myocardium.

Stimulation of noradrenergic nerves or injection of norepinephrine in unanaesthetised animals elicits coronary as vasoconstriction after administration of β-adrenergic blocking drug, that blocks the inotropic and chronotropic effects. Stimulation of vagal fibres to the heart causes coronary dilation.

MEASUREMENT OF CORONARY BLOOD FLOW

1. *Kety method*: Nitrous oxide method based on Fick's principle.
2. *Radionuclides*: Thallium 201 (^{201}Tl) has been used to study the regional blood flow in the heart, to detect areas of ischaemia and infarct, and also to evaluate ventricular functions. It is pumped into cardiac muscle cells by $Na^+ - K^+$ ATPase and equilibrates with intracellular K^+ pool. Thallium 201 distribution is directly proportional to the myocardial blood flow. Ischaemic areas have low uptake. The uptake of this radionuclide is diminished after exercise, as blood flow is compromised after exertion.
3. *Radiopharmaceuticals* such as technetium 99m stannous pyrophosphate (^{99m}Tc-PYP) are taken up by infarcted tissue in a selective manner. The infarcts can be detected as hot spots on scintiscans of the chest.
4. *Coronary angiography* is done by first injecting radio-opaque contrast medium and working out the details of coronary arteries with X-rays. This is combined with measurement of ^{133}Xe washout technique. This radioactive substance is

injected into left main coronary artery and the flow values for various regions under each scintillation detector are determined.

5. *Digital subtraction angiography (DSA):* Radio-opaque dye is injected. Imaging is done with an angioscope. A computer measures the degree of constriction of coronary arteries by converting the image into digital code and comparing it to others made from different angles. It also measures the rate at which blood diffuses into the heart muscle, i.e. whether or not a heart attack is likely to occur.

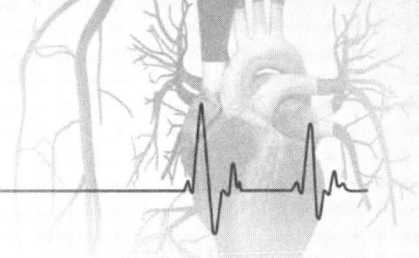

18

Cerebral Blood Flow

NORMAL VALUES

Normal blood flow through the brain tissue of adult averages 50–65 ml/100 gm/min (54 ml/100 gm/min). For entire brain, it is 750–900 ml/min (756 ml/min) or 15 per cent of the total resting cardiac output (for 1400 gm brain weight).

REGULATION OF CEREBRAL BLOOD FLOW

Constant cerebral blood flow is generally maintained under varying conditions. Despite extensive shifts in pattern of flow, total cerebral blood flow is not increased by strenuous mental activity.

Factors affecting the total cerebral blood flow
1. The mean arterial pressure at brain level
2. The mean venous pressure at brain level
3. The intracranial pressure
4. The viscosity of blood
5. The degree of active constriction or dilation of the cerebral arterioles

Caliber of the vessels is controlled by
1. Local vasodilator metabolites.
2. Autoregulation.
3. Locally acting substances produced by the endothelium, e.g. nitric oxide, endothelin.

4. Circulating peptides such as angiotensin II and substances released from the nerve endings.
5. Sympathetic post-ganglionic (releasing norepinephrine, neuropeptide-Y, etc.) and cholinergic neurons (acetylcholine, VIP) and sensory nerves (VIP, substance P, CGRP, neurokinin A).

Metabolic factors which have potent effects in controlling cerebral blood flow
• Carbon dioxide concentration
• Hydrogen ion concentration
• Oxygen concentration

An increase in either CO_2 or hydrogen ion concentration or decrease in oxygen concentration results in ↑ cerebral blood flow.

Regulation of cerebral blood flow in response to excess CO_2 or hydrogen ion concentration: A 70 per cent ↑ in CO_2 concentration in arterial blood increases the cerebral blood flow twice.

CO_2 combines with H_2O → carbonic acid → dissociates to form hydrogen ions → vasodilation.

Other acidic substances like lactic acid and pyruvic acid also ↑ blood flow.

Influence of carbon dioxide and hydrogen ions on cerebral blood flow: Increase in hydrogen ion concentration greatly depresses neuronal activity. Thus ↑ in hydrogen ion concentration → ↑ blood flow → CO_2, H^+ and other acidic substances are washed away from brain tissues.

Role of O_2 on cerebral blood flow: The utilisation of O_2 by brain tissue remains almost constant within 3.5 ml/100 gm/min. If the blood flow becomes insufficient, the O_2 deficiency causes vasodilation. A decrease in cerebral tissue PO_2 to less than 30 mmHg will immediately begin to increase cerebral blood flow.

AUTOREGULATION

In the arterial pressure range of 60–140 mmHg, there is not much change in the cerebral blood flow. In hypertensives, the upper

→ leads to; ↑ increase

limit shifts even to 180 mmHg. But below 60 mmHg, cerebral blood flow becomes severely compromised. Above 180 mmHg, it can cause severe rupture of cerebral blood vessels, resulting in serious brain oedema or cerebral haemorrhage.

ROLE OF SYMPATHETIC NERVOUS SYSTEM

There is strong sympathetic innervation from superior cervical sympathetic ganglia. However, the blood flow autoregulation mechanism can override the nervous effect.

With strenuous exercise, when arterial pressure rises high, sympathetic nervous system becomes activated and constricts the blood vessels (large and intermediate sized arteries) to prevent damage of smaller vessels.

EFFECT OF CEREBRAL ACTIVITY ON BLOOD FLOW

Blood flow in each individual segment of the brain changes within seconds in response to changes in local neuronal activity. However, it takes a few hundred milliseconds to a few seconds.

Making fist of the hand: Increase in the blood flow occurs in the motor cortex of the opposite side of the brain, in the hand area.

Reading the book: Blood flow increases in occipital cortex and language perception areas of the temporal cortex.

EFFECT OF INTRACRANIAL PRESSURE ON BLOOD FLOW

The brain, spinal cord and spinal fluid are encased along with the cerebral vessels in a rigid bony enclosure (1400 gm brain, 75 ml blood, 75 ml spinal fluid). As brain and spinal fluid are incompressible, the volume of blood, spinal fluid and brain in the cranium, at any time must be relatively constant ("Monro-Kellie doctrine"). When the intracranial pressure increases, the cerebral vessels are compressed.

When venous pressure increases, the intracranial pressure increases. This results in:
1. Compression of cerebral vessels
2. Decrease in the effective perfusion pressure
3. Decrease in blood flow.

CEREBRAL VASCULAR RESISTANCE (CVR)

Cerebral vascular resistance is defined as the *cerebral perfusion pressure* (cerebral arteriovenous difference) divided by *cerebral blood flow.*

$$CVR = \frac{\text{Cerebral perfusion pressure}}{\text{Cerebral blood flow}}$$

In supine position, mean brachial artery pressure is taken as cerebral perfusion pressure, ignoring the relatively low cerebral venous pressure. CVR is 7.2 R units for whole brain.

METHODS OF DETERMINATION OF CEREBRAL BLOOD FLOW

1. Kety Method

Inhaled nitrous oxide is used.

According to Fick's principle,

$$\text{Cerebral blood flow (CBF)} = \frac{Q_x}{(A_x - V_x)}$$

where Q_x is the amount of N_2O inhaled and $(A_x - V_x)$ is the cerebral arteriovenous difference.

Average cerebral blood in young adults is 54 ml/100 gm/min. Average adult brain weighs 1400 gm. Thus flow for the whole brain is 756 ml/min by this method.

Kety method gives an average value.

1. It does not measure regional differences in blood flow.
2. As it depends on N_2O uptake, it measures flow to perfused parts of brain only. The non-perfused areas do not take up any N_2O (nitrous oxide)

2. Recent Techniques for Monitoring Local Cerebral Blood Flow in Living Animals and Humans

Distribution of ^{133}Xe, [123] I-labelled iodoamphetamine or other tracers can be measured. The arrival and clearance of the tracer are monitored by a battery of scintillation detectors placed over the head. Output from the detectors is processed in a computer and displayed on a colour television screen. The colour is proportionate to the flow it is detecting. Resolution is improved with computerised tomographic reconstruction as is used in CT. This technique is called *single photon emission computed tomography* (SPECT).

3. Positron Emission Tomography (PET)

Blood flow is tightly coupled to metabolism. Blood flow increases with neuronal activity. Local uptake of 2-deoxyglucose, labelled with a short half-life positron emitter such as ^{18}F, ^{11}O or ^{15}O can be monitored by *positron emission tomography*, through intact skull in living subjects. Positrons combine with electrons to emit γ rays. The arrival and clearance of the tracer are monitored by scintillation detectors, connected to computer and television monitor, that displays the output of the detector as a particular colour, proportionate to the flow it is detecting.

4. Magnetic Resonance Imaging (MRI)

Localised changes in blood flow are monitored.

Functional magnetic resonance imaging (fMRI):

Regional concentration of individual metabolites can be measured and changes in local O_2 utilisation can be mapped by fMRI. The resolution is better than that of PET.

In resting humans, the blood flow of gray matter is 69 ml/ 100 gm/min and white matter is 28 ml/100 gm/min.

In subjects who are awake but at rest, flow is greatest in premotor and frontal region, which is decoding and analysing afferent input. It is also increased in these areas with intellectual activity. During voluntary contraction of a particular part, flow is increased in the opposite side motor cortex concerned with that area and corresponding sensory area.

With sequential movements flow is increased in the supplementary motor area. When subjects talk and speech is stereotyped there is bilateral increase in blood flow in the sensory and motor areas of face, tongue and mouth and upper premotor cortex in the categorical hemisphere (left). With creative speech, Broca's and Wernicke's areas show increased flow. With problem solving, reasoning and motor ideation without movement , flow increases in selected areas of premotor and frontal cortex.

Right-handed individuals: Blood flow to left hemisphere is greater when a verbal task is being performed and the blood flow to the right hemisphere is greater when spatial task is being performed. Blood flow to many brain areas, that are to be activated during the particular task, increases much before the activity.

SPECT, PET and fMRI

All these techniques can be used for the study of various diseases, epileptic foci, etc.

1. Epileptic foci have ↑ blood flow during seizures. Between seizures, the blood flow is decreased.
2. Parieto-occipital flow is decreased in patients with agnosia.
3. *Alzheimer's disease:* There is ↓ metabolism and blood flow in superior parietal cortex, which later spreads to temporal lobe and frontal cortex.
4. *Huntington's disease:* Bilateral reduction in blood flow to caudate nucleus.
5. *In depressives and schizophrenics:* There is decreased blood flow in frontal, temporal lobes and basal ganglia. During *aura* in patients with *migraine,* decrease in blood flow occurs in occipital cortex that spreads to temporal and parietal lobes.

↑ increase; ↓ decrease

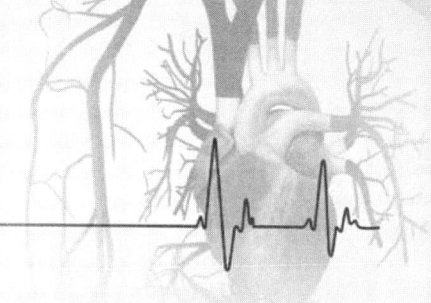

19

Circulation through the Skin

GENERAL FEATURES

1. Skin is the place from which reactions of blood vessels can be observed.
2. It regulates the amount of heat lost from the body by regulating its blood flow, which can vary from 1 to 150 ml/100 gm/min. The subdermal capillaries, the venous plexus and the arteriovenous anastomoses of fingers, toes, palms and earlobes are well innervated.

White Reaction

When a pointed object is drawn over the skin, lightly, the stroke lines become pale. In about 15 seconds, the mechanical stimulus initiates contraction of precapillary sphincters. In response to this, blood drains out of the capillaries and small veins.

Triple Response

Stroking of the skin more firmly with the pointed instrument results in three phenomena.

Red reaction: There is reddening at the site that appears in 10 seconds. The initial redness (red reaction) is due to capillary dilation.

Wheal: The read reaction is followed in a few minutes by local swelling and diffused mottled reddening around the injury. The swelling (wheal) is due to local oedema due to increase

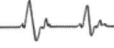

in permeability of capillaries and postcapillary venules, with extravasation of fluid.

Redness (flare): The diffuse, mottled, reddening around the injury that follows *red reaction* is known as *flare*. Flare is due to arteriolar dilation. Flare is absent in locally anaesthetised skin and in denervated skin after sensory nerves have degenerated. It is present above the site of injury after nerve section or block.

This three part response is known as *triple response*.

AXON REFLEX

Antidromic Conduction

Axon reflex is the physiological example of antidromic conduction. Impulses originated in the sensory nerve are relayed antidromically, down other sensory fibres to the arterioles.

Substance P is released by the afferent sensory C fibre neurons. CGRP also is present in neurons. Both the substances dilate arterioles.

During the wheal formation, histamine is released from mast cells and acts via H_1 receptors. Substance P also causes extravasation of fluid.

REACTIVE HYPERAEMIA

The other reaction visible in skin is *reactive hyperaemia*. After a period of occlusion, an ↑ in blood flow occurs in a region when its circulation is re-established. When blood supply is occluded, the arterioles below the occlusion dilate. When circulation is re-established, blood flowing into dilated vessels causes the skin to become fiery red. It is due to local effect of hypoxia. It can be prevented, if the artery is blocked in 100% O_2 atmosphere.

General Responses

Noradrenergic nerve stimulation and circulating epinephrine and norepinephrine constrict cutaneous blood vessels. Vasodilation is brought about by decrease in vasoconstrictor tone and there are no vasodilator fibres, vasodilation is also brought about by vasodilator metabolites and in sweat glands by bradykinin.

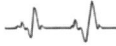

Other Reactions of Skin

Constriction of arterioles and dilation of capillaries result in a cold blue or gray skin. When arterioles and capillaries are dilated, the skin is warm and red. When there is increase in hypothalamic temperature due to exercise, etc., dilation of cutaneous vessels occurs.

Cold causes cutaneous vasoconstriction. With severe cold, superficial vasodilation occurs.

Muscle Blood Flow

NORMAL VALUES

The blood flow of resting skeletal muscle is 3–4 ml/min/ 100 gm of muscle. During strenuous exercise, muscle blood flow increases to 15–25 times, i.e. 45–80 ml/min/100 gm to supply O_2 and essential nutrients to muscles and to remove metabolic waste products. During rhythmical contractions, the flow decreases or even ceases during each contraction as:

1. The contracting muscle compresses the intramuscular blood vessels
2. Strong tetanic muscle contractions can cause rapid muscle fatigue. Due to sustained muscle contraction, delivery of nutrients and O_2 to contracting muscle is severely compromised. When a muscle develops more than 70 per cent of its maximal tension, blood flow is completely stopped. However, in between the rhythmical contractions, blood flow increases as much as 30 times.

CIRCULATORY ADJUSTMENTS TO EXERCISE

Local Mechanisms (Table 20.1)

Almost half of the increase in flow results from intramuscular vasodilation caused by increased muscle metabolism, release of chemical vasodilator substances and decreased O_2 and nutrient concentration.

Table 20.1: Local mechanisms that control blood flow during exercise

Local change during exercise	Physiological effect
1. ↓ in PO_2, ↑ in PCO_2, ↑ temperature, ↑ K^+, ↑ vasodilator metabolites	Dilation of the arterioles, opening up of new capillaries, ↑ in the cross-sectional area of vascular bed, ↓ velocity of blood flow, ↑ capillary pressure exceeding oncotic pressure, favouring fluid transudation
2. ↓ pH, ↑ temperature, ↑ concentration of 2, 3-DPG in red cells	O_2 dissociation curve for haemoglobin shifts to right, making more oxygen available
3. Accumulation of osmotically active substances	↓ osmotic gradient across capillaries, ↑ fluid transudation into interstitial spaces, ↑ lymph flow
4. Muscles use more O_2	↓ tissue PO_2 and venous PO_2→ ↑ arteriovenous difference → better extraction of oxygen by tissues, facilitation of CO_2 transport

↑ increased; ↓ decreased; → leads to

Systemic Changes

The motor areas of the cerebral cortex not only send signals to the muscles to be activated for performing the exercise, but also send impulses to the vasomotor centre, initiating *mass sympathetic discharge*. There is vasoconstriction of the small arteries and arterioles, increasing the total peripheral resistance and arterial pressure. Venoconstriction causes translocation of blood towards the heart, increasing venous return. Increase in heart rate and force of contraction cause increase in cardiac output. At the same time, parasympathetic impulses to the heart are inhibited.

Moderate increase in arterial pressure not only pushes more blood through the vessels, but also stretches the walls of the arterioles and further reduces the vascular resistance. Blood flow sometimes increases at or even before the start of exercise. This is neurally mediated and the sympathetic vasodilator system may be involved. During rest, some of the muscle capillaries are not open. With strenuous exercise, the dormant capillaries open, blood flows through these capillaries, reducing the distance for diffusion of O_2, CO_2 and nutrients back and forth between muscle tissue and blood vessels.

ISOMETRIC EXERCISE

1. ↑ heart rate (psychic stimuli, ↓ vagal tone, ↑ discharge of cardiac sympathetic nerves)
2. ↑ systolic blood pressure, and ↑ diastolic blood pressure occur simultaneously
3. Stroke volume does not change much
4. ↑ peripheral resistance resulting from sustained contraction of muscles and ↓ muscle blood flow
5. External work is not done

ISOTONIC EXERCISE

1. ↑ heart rate
2. ↑ systolic blood pressure (moderate)
3. ↓ diastolic blood pressure or no change, due to vasodilation
4. ↑ stroke volume (marked)
5. ↓ peripheral resistance
6. ↑ cardiac output to 35 L/min, proportionate to ↑ in O_2 consumption, and work done by exercising muscles
7. ↑ venous return → Due to ↑ activity in muscle and thoracic pumps
   → Mobilisation of blood from viscera
   → Venoconstriction

TEMPERATURE REGULATION DURING EXERCISE

1. Warm muscle blood → transported to skin → heat lost/radiated to environment
2. ↑ Ventilation → heat lost in expired air
3. ↑ Body temperature → hypothalamic sensors → heat dissipating mechanisms activated
4. Sweat secretion → heat lost through evaporation.

The temperature increase occurs, when the above heat dissipating mechanisms are unable to handle the heat load.

→ leads to; ↑ increase; ↑ decrease

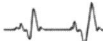

WORK OUTPUT, OXYGEN CONSUMPTION AND CARDIAC OUTPUT DURING EXERCISE

O_2 Consumption during Exercise and O_2 Debt

The oxygen consumption, the muscle blood flow and the cardiac output all increase proportionately and the energy needs are supplied by the aerobic pathway up to certain point.

Replenishment of energy stores, i.e. ATP and phosphoryl creatine is by $\to$ aerobic breakdown of free fatty acids (FFA), glycogen and glucose to $\to CO_2$ and H_2O.

When the muscular exercise is very severe and the energy demands of the muscles exceed the aerobic resynthesis of energy stores, ATP is synthesised through anaerobic pathway, by breakdown of glucose or glycogen to lactate.

Thus, when exercise is severe and for short duration$\to\uparrow$ in O_2 consumption is unable to meet tissue demands $\to O_2$ debt is incurred $\to$ breakdown of carbohydrates to pyruvate and then anaerobically to lactate occurs.

O_2 consumption remains high even after exercise, till the O_2 debt is paid off.

EFFECT OF TRAINING

With training, the heart chambers and the heart muscle hypertrophy (40%) in marathoners. The resting cardiac output is same and is achieved by an increase in stroke volume and $\downarrow$ in heart rate.

Cardiac output at various levels of exercise:	Litres/min
Average young man at rest	5.5 l/min
Maximum average output during exercise, in young untrained man	25 l/min
Maximum average output during exercise, in male marathoner	30–35 l/min

Trainees: Have $\uparrow$ muscle glycogen
              Utilise FFA more effectively
              So have $\downarrow$ lactate production.

$\to$ leads to; $\uparrow$, increase; $\downarrow$ decrease

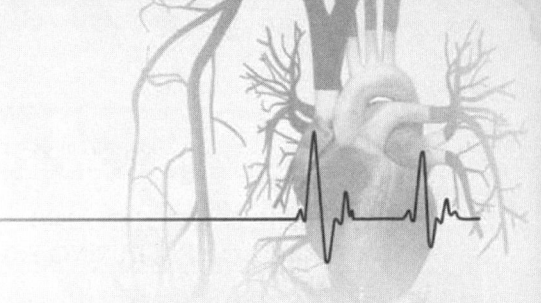

Cardiac Failure

DEFINITION

Cardiac failure is defined as the failure of the heart to pump enough blood, to satisfy the needs of the body.

Causes

1. Pathological conditions of the heart that reduce the ability of the heart to pump blood, due to decrease in coronary blood flow (myocardial infarction), hypertension known as *forward failure, left heart failure* or *systolic failure*.
2. Damaged heart valves, valvular heart disease, e.g.
   a. Mitral or aortic valve stenosis—resulting in left heart failure
   b. Tricuspid or pulmonary stenosis or right heart disease resulting in *right heart failure, backward failure, congestive heart failure*.
3. External pressure around the heart: Pericarditis, pericardial effusion
4. Primary cardiac muscle disease can involve left or right side or both, e.g. cardiac myopathies.
5. Increased demand of the tissues, i.e. *high output failure*, e.g. thiamine deficiency, thyrotoxicosis, large arteriovenous fistula, anaemia, fever, etc.

SYSTOLIC HEART FAILURE

- Stroke volume is reduced as ventricular contractions are weak.
- End-systolic volume increases, ejection fraction decreases.
- Salt and water retention occur due to compensatory phenomena.

DIASTOLIC HEART FAILURE

- Cardiac filling is defective, as there is resistance to filling due to loss of elasticity.
- Stroke volume decreases, ejection fraction decreases.
- Salt and water retention occur. Heart failure commonly involves the left ventricle but can involve the right ventricle also *cor pulmonale.*

ACUTE CARDIAC FAILURE

Sudden onset

CHRONIC CARDIAC FAILURE

Due to gradual deterioration of heart function.

Compensatory Mechanisms for Acute Cardiac Failure

At first, cardiac output is only decreased during exercise and remains normal during rest. As the disease progresses, it becomes evident even at rest. When the cardiac output falls low, many of the sympathetic reflexes get activated.

The low output initiates the baroreceptor reflex. There is generalized vasoconstriction, including vasoconstriction in the kidneys. Renin is released and aldosterone is secreted leading to increased retention of fluid and Na^+. In addition to these physiological compensatory mechanisms, the chemoreceptor reflex, the central nervous system ischaemic response and the reflexes that originate in the damaged heart contribute to activating sympathetic nervous system.

The sympathetic reflexes give time to the hypoeffective heart for recovery and within seconds initiate other compensatory mechanisms like:

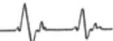

1. Stimulating the functional cardiac muscle and making it a stronger pump.
2. Increasing the contraction of veins, thus increasing mean systemic filling pressure.

Chronic State of Cardiac Failure

After acute heart attack, the chronic state sets in. It is characterized by retention of fluid by the kidneys and varying degrees of recovery of the heart over weeks to months.

1. *Fluid retention*: Decreased cardiac output and increased sympathetic discharge result in decreased renal output and fluid retention. Moderate fluid retention is beneficial as this reconstitutes the blood volume and increases mean systemic filling pressure, thus increasing the venous return to the heart. However, severe failure and excess of fluid retention are detrimental.
2. Heart itself recovers slowly.

The manifestations of heart failure range from sudden death through cardiogenic shock to chronic congestive heart failure. Often the systolic dysfunction is denoted as forward failure due to forward failure of left ventricle, as the cardiac output is not sufficient for the exercising muscles, thus causing weakness specially during exercise.

Diastolic dysfunction is denoted as backward failure.

The major clinical features of congestive heart failure/backward failure: Backward failure sets in due to ineffective pumping, increased endsystolic volume or resistance to filling during diastole. The peripheral venous pressure increases, causing fluid transudation and ankle and sacral oedema. Hepatomegaly, pulmonary congestion, dyspnoea on exertion and cardiac dilation are other clinical features.

Decompensated Failure

Heart fails to pump out enough cardiac output for the normal renal excretion of salt and water and there is excess fluid retention, oedema, and eventually death.

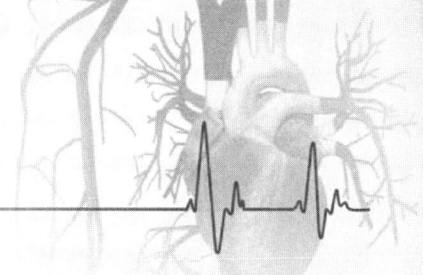

22

Cardiovascular Homeostasis

GRAVITATIONAL EFFECTS

Gravitational changes can be classified under the following headings:
1. Change in posture from recumbent to standing
2. Prolonged standing
3. Effects of acceleration—*positive 'g', negative 'g'* and *zero gravity.*

The following normal physiological data are to be noted:
- Mean arterial blood pressure in the feet of a normal adult is 180–200 mmHg and venous pressure is 85–90 mmHg in standing position.
- The arterial pressure at head level is 60–75 mmHg and venous pressure is 0 mmHg.
- While standing, 300–500 ml of blood pools in the venous capacitance vessels of lower extremities, if the individual dose not move. Fluid moves into interstitial spaces and stroke volume decreases.
- Symptoms of cerebral ischaemia develop, if cerebral blood flow is less than 60% of the flow in recumbent position.
- On assuming the upright posture, the fall in the blood pressure elicits baroreceptor reflex from the carotid sinus and aortic arch, leading to mass sympathetic discharge.

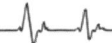

This results in:
1. ↑ Heart rate which causes increase in cardiac output
2. Venoconstriction that results in—translocation of blood towards heart, ↑ mean systemic filling pressure, ↑ in venous return
3. Arteriolar constriction that results in—↑ total peripheral resistance and ↑ in arterial pressure.
4. ↑ in circulating levels of renin and aldosterone—↑ fluid and ↑ Na^+ absorption, blood volume resuscitated.

The cerebral blood flow is not affected much as drop in arterial pressure at head level of 20–40 mmHg leads to ↓ in jugular venous pressure of 5–8 mmHg, thus compensating for the drop in arterial pressure that otherwise might have resulted in drop in perfusion pressure (arterial pressure–venous pressure). Decrease in intracranial pressure reduces the cerebral vascular resistance and facilitates blood flow.

↑ PCO_2, ↓ PO_2 and ↓ pH in brain tissue cause vasodilation of the cerebral blood vessels, thus maintaining the cerebral blood flow on standing. In addition, O_2 extraction increases.

Prolonged standing, e.g. in military personnel, standing at attention for long periods →↑ interstitial fluid volume in lower extremities → when the cerebral blood flow decreases to less than 60 per cent, the individual faints → it is a compensatory mechanism to make the person assume recumbent posture.

On the other hand, when the individual moves about → the muscle pump operates → keeps the venous pressure <30 mmHg in the feet.

Effect of gravity is more, if blood volume is low.

POSTURAL HYPOTENSION OR ORTHOSTATIC HYPOTENSION (Fig. 22.1)

Causes
1. Patients receiving sympatholytic drugs
2. Damage to sympathetic neurons, e.g. diabetes, syphilis

↑ increased; ↓ decreased; → leads to

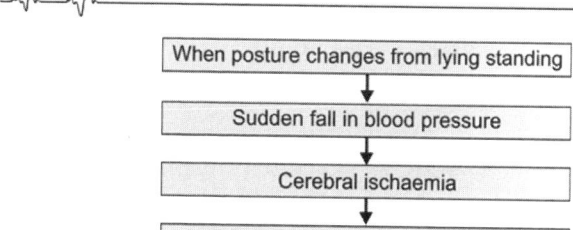

Fig. 22.1: Postural hypotension or orthostatic hypotension

3. Primary autonomic failure:
    i. Bradbury-Eggleston syndrome (idiopathic orthostatic hypotension)
    ii. Shy-Drager syndrome (multiple system atrophy)
    iii. Riley-Day syndrome (familial dysautonomia)
    iv. Dopamine β-hydroxylase deficiency
4. Primary hyperaldosteronism: Baroreceptor reflexes are abnormal. However, due to increase in blood volume, this effect is not evident.

EFFECTS OF ACCELERATION

- Expressed in g units, 1g is the force of gravity on the earths' surface that acts on body.
- *Positive g* is the force due to acceleration, acting in the long axis of the body, i.e. from head to foot, resulting in pooling of blood in lower extremities (Fig. 22.2).
- *Negative g* is the force due to deceleration, acting in the opposite direction, i.e. from foot to head, throwing blood upwards to the head and neck (Fig. 22.3).
- At acceleration of >5 g, vision fails in about 5 seconds and unconsciousness occurs.
- The effects of positive g can be countered by the use of antigravity "g" suits.

Intense congestion of head and neck vessels, etc. mental confusion (red out) occurs: Humans can tolerate 11 g acting in a back to chest direction for 3 minutes and 17 g acting in a chest to back direction.

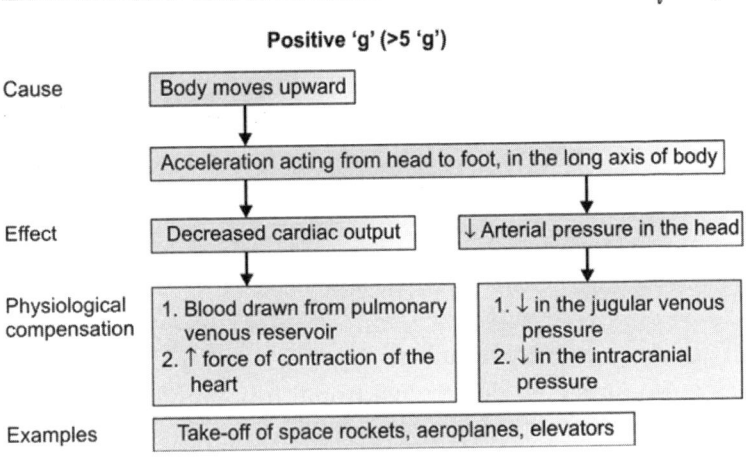

Fig. 22.2: Physiological effects of positive 'g' and compensation

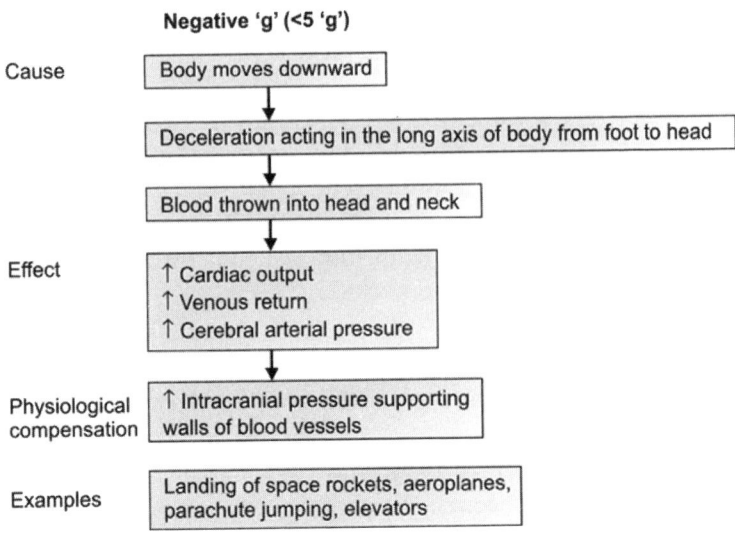

Fig. 22.3: Physiological effects of negative 'g' and compensation

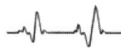

EFFECTS OF ZERO GRAVITY (Fig. 22.4)

Cause	Absence of earth's gravitational effect, zero gravity
	↓
	Weightlessness, body movements become effortless. Absence of hydrostatic pressure on the blood column
Effects	1. Transient postural hypotension
	4–7 weeks for readaptation after return from orbital flights
	2. Atrophy of myocardium, disuse atrophy of the heart, cardiovascular and somatic reflex mechanism responsible for postural adjustments.
	3. ↓ muscular effort →↓ in proprioceptive impulses → flaccidity and atrophy of skeletal muscles
	4. Space motion sickness
	5. Loss of plasma volume → due to headward shift of body fluids → subsequent diuresis
	6. Loss of muscle mass
	7. Steady loss of Ca^{2+} (bone mineral)
	8. Loss of red cell mass
	9. Psychological problems associated with isolation and monotony
Example	When astronauts in a spacecraft take orbital flights to other planets

Fig. 22.4: Effects of zero gravity (→ leads to; ↓ decrease)

Bibliography

1. Berne and Levy. Principles of Physiology, fourth edition, Editors, Bruce M Koeppen Mathew, N Levy and Bruce A Stanton, Associate Editors, Elsevier Mossby Publications, 2006.
2. Review of Medical Physiology. William F Ganong, twenty-second edition, McGraw-Hill Companies Inc, 2005.
3. Textbook of Medical Physiology. Arthur C Guyton and John E Hall, eleventh edition, Elsevier Publications, 2006.
4. Textbook of Medical Physiology. Indu Khurana, Elsevier Publications, 2006.

Index

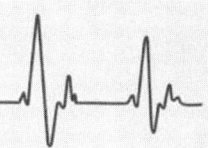

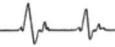

CHAPTER 19

SOME TYPICAL EXAMINATION QUESTIONS IN PRACTICAL

I.   1. Assay the given boric acid solution and report the content of boric acid in % w/v. You are provided with standard normal oxalic acid solution.

(Standardise the given approximately normal sodium hydroxide solution by using the standard oxalic acid solution and then assay the boric acid solution using the standard sodium hydroxide solution).

2. Perform the limit test for chlorides on the given sample of Dextrose, I.P. and report on its standard.

3. Perform the identification tests on the given sample of Sodium Bicarbonate, I.P. and report on its identity.

II.   1. Assay the given sample of hydrogen peroxide solution and report the content of hydrogen peroxide in % w/v. You are provided with a standard decinormal solution of oxalic acid.

(Standardise the given approximately decinormal potassium permanganate solution with standard oxalic acid solution. Then assay the hydrogen peroxide solution using the standard potassium permanganate solution).

2. Carry out the limit test for sulphates on the given sample of Citric Acid, I.P. and report on its standard.

3. Perform the identification tests on the given sample of Dicalcium Phosphate, I.P. and report on its identity.

III.   1. Assay the given iodine solution and report the content of iodine in % w/v. You are provided with standard decinormal potassium dichromate solution.

(Standardise the given approximately decinormal sodium thiosulphate solution by the use of standard decinormal potassium dichromate solution. Then assay the iodine solution using the standard sodium thiosulphate solution).

2. Perform the limit test for iron on the given sample of Sodium Chloride, I.P. and report on its standard.

3. Perform the identification tests on the given sample of Zinc Sulphate, I.P and report on its identity.

Some More Typical Assay Questions
Acidimetry - Alkalimetry

1. Assay the given sample of sodium bicarbonate solution and report on the content of sodium bicarbonate in % w/v. You are provided with standard $\frac{N}{2}$ sodium hydroxide solution. (Standardise $\frac{N}{2}$ sulphuric acid with standard $\frac{N}{2}$ sodium hydroxide solution and use the acid for assay of sodium bicarbonate).

2. Assay the given sample of ammonium chloride solution and report on its content in % w/v. You are provided with standard decinormal oxalic acid solution.

   (Standardise the given sodium hydroxide solution with standard oxalic acid solution and use it for assaying the ammonium chloride solution).

Permanganimetry

3. Assay the given ferrous sulphate solution and report on its content in % w/v. You are provided with an approximately decinormal potassium permanganate solution.

   (Standardise the potassium permanganate solution with standard decinormal oxalic acid solution and use it for assaying the ferrous sulphate solution).

Iodometry

4. Assay the given sample of Chlorinated Lime, I.P. and report on its standard. You are provided with an approximately decinormal sodium thiosulphate solution.

(Standardise the sodium thiosulphate solution with standard decinormal potassium dichromate solution and use it for assaying the chlorinated lime. If the content of available chlorine is determined to be more than 30% w/v, declare the sample as standard. If it is below 30% w/v, then declare the sample as substandard).

Argentimetry

5. Assay the given sample of Sodium Chloride Injection, I.P. and report on its standard. You are provided with standard decinormal sodium chloride solution.

(Standardise the decinormal silver nitrate solution using the standard sodium chloride solution and also standardise the ammonium thiocyanate solution using the standard silver nitrate solution. Then assay the sodium chloride injection in the usual way using the standard silver nitrate and ammonium thiocyanate solutions -- modified Volhard's method. Then declare the injection to be standard or substandard as per limits given in the I.P.)

Complexometry

6. Assay the given sample of magnesium sulphate solution and report on its content in % w/v.

Assay by using the procedure given in the book.

7. Assay the given sample of calcium gluconate solution and report on its content in % w/v.

Assay by using the procedure given in the book.